J.L. Atlee · H. Gombotz · K.H. Tscheliessnigg (Eds.)

# Perioperative Management of Pacemaker Patients

With 37 Figures and 30 Tables

Springer-Verlag
Berlin Heidelberg New York London Paris Tokyo
HongKong Barcelona Budapest

Prof. Dr. J.L. Atlee III
Dept. of Anesthesiology
Miwaukee Country Medical Complex
8700 West Wisconsin Avenue
Milwaukee, WI 53226, USA

Univ. Doz. Dr. H. Gombotz
Klinik für Anästhesiologie
Landeskrankenhaus Graz
Auenbruggerplatz 29
A-8036 Graz, Österreich

Prof. Dr. K.H. Tscheliessnigg
Abt. für Transplantationschirurgie
Universitätsklinik für Chirurgie
Auenbruggerplatz 29
A-8036 Graz, Österreich

ISBN 3-540-53874-7 Springer Verlag Berlin Heidelberg New York
ISBN 0-387-53874-7 Springer Verlag New York Berlin Heidelberg


Printed in Germany

*Product Liability:* The publisher can give no guarantee for information about drug dosage and application thereof contained in this book. In every individual case the respective user must check its accuracy by consulting other pharmaceutical literature.
The use of registered names, trademarks, etc. in this publication does not imply, even in the absence of a specific statement, that such names are exempt from the relevant protective laws and regulations and therefore free for general use.

Typesetting: Fotosatz & Design Reiter, Berchtesgaden
2119/3130-543210 – Printed on acid-free paper

# Contents

# Contributors

Anelli-Monti M., Department of Surgery, University of Graz, Auenbruggerplatz 29, A–8036 LKH-Graz, Austria

Arian-Schad K., Department of Radiotherapy, University of Graz, Auenbruggerplatz 29, A-8036 LKH-Graz, Austria

Atlee III, J.L., Department of Anesthesiology, Medical College of Wisconsin, Milwaukee County Medical Complex, 8700 West Wisconsin Avenue, Milwaukee, WI 53226, USA

Beitzke A., Department of Pediatric Cardiology, Department of Pediatrics, University of Graz, Auenbruggerplatz, A-8036 LKH-Graz, Austria

Bossert T., Institut für Rundfunktechnik, Floriansmühle 60, W-8000 München, FRG

Bourgeois I.M.G.P., Bakken Research Center, Endepolsdomein 5, 6229 GW, Maastricht, The Netherlands

Brouwer H., Vitatron Medical B.V., Reigerstraat 30, 6883 ES, Velp, The Netherlands

Chapman P.D., Department of Cardiology-Hypertension, Medical College of Wisconsin, Milwaukee County Medical Complex, 8700 West Wisconsin Avenue, Milwaukee, WI 53226, USA

Dacar D., Department of Surgery, University of Graz, Auenbruggerplatz 29, A-8036 LKH-Graz, Austria

Gleissner M., Hofaue 93, W-5600 Wuppertal, FRG

Gombotz H., Department of Anesthesiology, University of Graz, Auenbruggerplatz 29, A-8036 LKH-Graz, Austria

Hedman A.G., Department of Medicine, Ludvika Hospital, Ludvika S-77181, Sweden

Hove van J.W.J., Vitatron Medical B.V., Reigerstraat 30, 6883 ES, Velp, The Netherlands

Iberer F., Department of Surgery, University of Graz, Auenbruggerplatz 29, A-8036 LKH-Graz, Austria

Irnich W., Institut für Medizinische Technik, Justus-Liebig-Universität, Aulweg 123, W-6300 Gießen, FRG

Justich E., Department of Radiology, University of Graz, Auenbruggerplatz, A-8036 LKH-Graz, Austria

Klein W., Division of Cardiology, Department of Medicine, University of Graz, Auenbruggerplatz, A-8036 LKH-Graz, Austria

Lazica M., Urologische Abteilung, Klinikum Barmen, W-5600 Wuppertal-Barmen, FRG

Leitgeb N., Department for Clinical Engineering, Institute for Biomedical Engineering, Graz University of Technology, Inffeldgasse 18, A-8010 Graz, Austria

List W.F., Department of Anesthesiology, University of Graz, Auenbruggerplatz 29, A-8036 LKH-Graz, Austria

Mächler H. E., Department of Surgery, University of Graz, Auenbruggerplatz 29, A-8036 LKH-Graz, Austria

Mahla E., Department of Anesthesiology, University of Graz, Auenbruggerplatz 29, A-8036 LKH-Graz, Austria

Metzler H., Department of Anesthesiology, University of Graz, Auenbruggerplatz 29, A-8036 LKH-Graz, Austria

Poier E., Department of Radiotherapy, University of Graz, Auenbruggerplatz 29, A-8036 LKH-Graz, Austria

Posch W., Institut für Bürgerliches Recht, Heinrichstr. 22, A-8010 Graz, Austria

Rotman B., Department of Cardiology, University of Graz, Auenbruggerplatz, A-8036 LKH-Graz, Austria

Schaldach M., Zentralinstitut für Biomedizinische Technik, Universität Erlangen, Turnstr. 5, W-8520 Erlangen, FRG

Schick P., Institut für Strafrecht, Strafprozeßrecht und Kriminologie, Universitätsstraße 27, A-8010 Graz, Austria

Sovinz P., Department of Pediatric Cardiology, Department of Pediatrics, University of Graz, Auenbruggerplatz, A-8036 LKH-Graz, Austria

Stein J.I., Department of Pediatric Cardiology, Department of Pediatrics, University of Graz, Auenbruggerplatz, A-8036 LKH-Graz, Austria

Sutton R., Westminster Hospital, Horse Ferry Road, London SW1P 2AP, UK

Tscheliessnigg K.H., Department of Surgery, University of Graz, Auenbruggerplatz 29, A-8036 LKH-Graz, Austria

Wasler A., Department of Surgery, University of Graz, Auenbruggerplatz 29, A-8036 LKH-Graz, Austria

# Preface

A symposium, „Perioperative Management of Pacemaker Patients“, was held in May 1990 at the Karl-Franzens-Universität, Landeskrankenhaus Graz, Austria. The purpose of the symposium, organized by the Departments of Anesthesiology and Surgery, was to discuss the current status of permanent pacemaker technology, emerging developments in this field, legal issues, indications and methods for temporary perioperative pacing, and the potential for pacemaker malfunction and adverse patient-pacemaker interactions in perioperative and other medical settings. It was hoped that participants would come to some consensus concerning recommendations for satisfactory perioperative management of pacemaker patients.

This symposium was probably the first occasion ever that brought together representatives of the pacemaker industry, implanting physicians, and physicians responsible for the management of pacemaker patients in perioperative and other hospital settings to discuss these important matters. Certainly, it was recognized by all who attended that there existed at the time little in the way of substantial knowledge of how to best manage pacemaker patients or patients with possible indications for temporary pacing in „unique“ hospital settings especially with exposure to electromagnetic and other potential interference, but in the absence of professional persons with direct knowledge of pacemakers and related devices. Much new information was presented and useful ideas exchanged, so that three symposium participants were of the opinion that papers presented at this meeting should be published as a collective work. Additional authors were recruited (not necessarily symposium participants) to provide chapters on topics not addressed at the symposium, but relevant to perioperative pacemaker management. This book, somewhat delayed in appearance on account of the time required for translation (from German) and editing of manuscripts, represents the culmination of these efforts.

The editors, two of whom are anesthesiologists and intensive care specialists (J.L.A., H.G.), and one an implanting physician (K.H.T.), asked each author to prepare a manuscript based on his presentation at the symposium held in Graz or a later-assigned topic. Manuscripts were edited, some more stringently than others, so that the collected work had some sense of organization around the theme of this book. Thus, initial chapters present an overview of existing pacemaker technology and ongoing or planned developments in this field. Two chapters follow, one of which presents one group's experience with pacemakers in infants and children and the other which describes implantable cardioverter defibrillators. The next five chapters address pacemaker malfunction due to electromagnetic and mechanical interference, radiofrequency transmission interference, nuclear magnetic resonance imaging, radiation therapy and extracorporeal shock wave lithotripsy and also provide the chapter author's recommendations for management of pacemaker patients exposed to any of these potential causes of pacemaker malfunction. Another chapter provides a legal perspective of existing and emerging pacemaker technology, including manufacturer's, distributor's and physician's obligations or responsibilities. Indications for permanent pacing are then presented, followed by chapters describing the place of temporary pacing in cardiopulmonary resuscitation and methods for preoperative assessment of patients with suspected bradycardiac arrhythmias. Separate chapters toward the end of the book discuss indications and methods for temporary perioperative pacing and specifically address the problem of pacemaker malfunction in perioperative settings. The final chapter, a summary of sorts and written after editing of all previous chapters, was prepared by the editors to be a concise reference for the types of pacemaker malfunction to expect in perioperative settings as well as to offer guidelines for preventive management.

Finally, the editors express their sincere appreciation to Ilse Gombotz for assisting with the English translations of manuscripts that were formerly in German and to Gudrun Gsell for secretarial assistance. Additionally we thank Claudia Osthoff of Springer-Verlag for enabling us to realize our goal of having the Graz symposium proceedings made available to all who are interested in the perioperative management of pacemaker patients, but who previously have had no ready access to pertinent, contemporary information.

The Editors

# Current Status of Pacemaker Technology

M. Schaldach

## Introduction

The sequence of contraction in the heart is controlled by autonomous mechanisms which are subject to extracardiac regulative influences [1–4]. Through sympathetic innervation, these mechanisms permit inotropic and chronotropic adaptation of the cardiac output to physical workload. The automatic action begins at the sinoatrial (SA) node. If SA impulse formation ceases or the impulse is blocked, e.g., SA block or total atrioventricular (AV) block, the remaining parts of the conduction system are capable of spontaneous excitation (secondary pacemakers). However, as the distance of the secondary pacemaker from the SA node increases, the rate of stimulus formation decreases. With secondary pacemakers, the workload-dependent variation in heart rate is also compromised, so that the cardiac output is regulated exclusively through changes in stroke volume. However, this compensatory mechanism presupposes a healthy ventricular myocardium for adapting the changes in stroke volume. In the event that this adaption does not compensate for the absence of increase in heart rate, bradycardiac symptoms can be successfully treated by implanting a permanent cardiac pacemaker [5–8]. For the workload-dependent adaptation of the cardiac output, augmented heart rate makes the largest contribution. This can be achieved by reestablishing physiological excitation with rate-adaptive, atrial-controlled pacing or by adaptation of the pacing rate through other physiological sensors, including corporeal, cardiovascular, hemodynamic, and metabolic parameters [8–16].

The multidisciplinary approach to technical solutions is based on the component aspects of the problem. The solution relies upon the physiological, physical, electrochemical, and material sciences. The engineering and scientific contributions entail not only signal processing, control engineering, and microelectronics, but also the incorporation of material sciences and process engineering. As with the solution of other problems in biomedical engineering, the development of cardiac pacemakers depends critically on the mastery of basic technologies. The reliability and safety of the technical therapeutic device requires comprehensive quality control measures which must include all of the system components. The multidisciplinary nature of engineering and scientific contributions to pacemaker technology is summarized in Figure 1.

By way of example, concerning pacemaker electrodes, processes at the electrode are characterized by the electrophysiological and electrochemical conditions at the electrode/myocardium phase boundary [17]. Pacemaker electronics make stringent

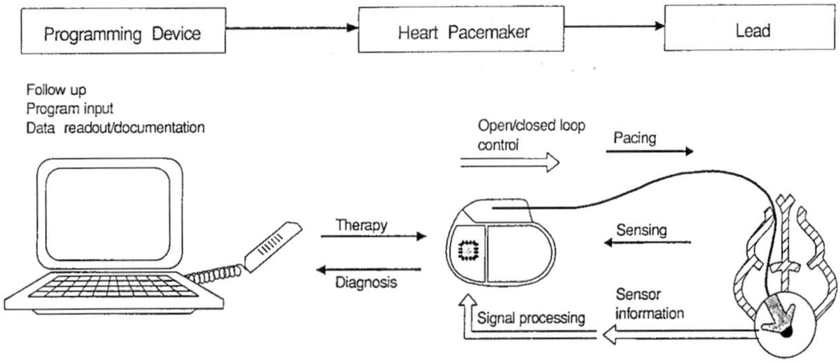


| Computer technology | Control system | Microelectronics | Processing technology | Materials research |
|---|---|---|---|---|
| • Hardware<br>• Software<br>• Modelling of biological Systems<br>• Signal transmission (digital/coded)<br>• Information processing | • Control technology<br>• Signal processing<br>• Information science<br>• Analog-/digital technology<br>• Sensor science<br>• Pathophysiology<br>• Cardiology<br>• Cybernetics | • VLSI, Low voltage<br>• RAM, ROM<br>• Microprocessor<br>• Hybrid technology | • Encapsulation<br>• (Electron-,laser-, plasma- beam welding)<br>• Metallurgy<br>• Polymer technology<br>• Insulation materials | • Electrophysiology<br>• Electrochemistry<br>• Biocompatibility<br>• Surface physics<br>• Polymer chemistry |

**Fig. 1.** Multidisciplinary nature of engineering and scientific contributions to pacemaker technology

demands on microelectronics with low power consumption. The microelectronics must not only serve for signal processing, but must also meet the control (stimulation) requirements of the device. Achieving an operating time matched to the life expectancy of the patient primarily depends on the power supply [18]. Experience has shown that other aspects, such as long-term stability of the insulating materials, minimizing of foreign body reactions (biocompatibility) and resistance to corrosion, also have a considerable influence on the trouble-free operation of the pacemaker. As the pacing devices have become more complex, bidirectional communication is required to manage the signal-processing and pacing modes of the device. The principle of the pacemaker is essentially based on a timer with a switching stage, with the timer being controlled by sensed cardiac activity. The energy necessary for artificial pacing is transferred to the myocardium from a storage capacitor. The subsequent repolarization process reestablishes charge neutrality, thus minimizing irreversible chemical reactions with a consequent rise in pacing thresholds [19, 20].

In today's pacemakers, interference between pacemaker stimulation and the heart's intrinsic rhythm is avoided by continuously monitoring the intracardiac electrogram (EGM). If cardiac activity remains absent for some predetermined interval, the pacemaker intervenes to reverse bradycardia or cardiac asystole. Such "demand" pacing is a feature of all modern single- and dual-chamber pacemakers.

The development of electrotherapy for cardiac rhythm disturbances is closely connected to our understanding of normal and abnormal cardiac electrophysiology, as well as the technical progress in electronic circuit, battery, and electrode technology. Technological progress has made it possible to produce pacemakers which will, in practice, accomplish most any therapeutic goal. Further, pacemakers are now reasonably sized while still providing a service life matched to the life expectancy of most patients.

## Implantable Pacemakers: History, Current Status, and Trends

The first artificial pacemaker was developed by Elmquist and implanted by Senning in 1958 [21]. Electrostimulation soon became the therapy of choice for bradycardic arrhythmias. The implantable pacemaker was made possible by the invention of the transistor. The circuit in the first pacemakers made use of a simple resistance capacitance (RC) element to control the pacing rate; however, early pacemakers did not monitor intrinsic cardiac activity (no demand function). Due to lack of demand function, termed asynchronous ventricular pacing (VOO), there was always the possibility of interference between the artificial pacemaker and spontaneous rhythm.

The next logical step (1960s) was the development of ventricular-triggered (VTT) and inhibited (VVI) pacemakers. Both devices necessitated the addition of an ECG amplifier and R-wave detection circuit. These pacemakers were built using discrete transistors, which limited achievable functionality. In the early 1970s, the incorporation of integrated circuits permitted the design of programmable units with greater functionality. Those devices allowed postoperative adjustment of many pacing parameters. Addition of programmability greatly facilitated the management of patients throughout the useful service time of the device. At about the same time, the introduction of the lithium iodine battery extended the operating time of the device to more nearly match the life expectancy of most patients.

Parallel to the efforts to enhance single-chamber devices, "physiological pacemakers" were developed. The first devices operated in the ventricular activation time (VAT) mode; that is, ventricular pacing was triggered by detected atrial electrical activity. For patients with AV block but intact sinus node function, these devices were a decisive step toward an improved quality of life. The next step was to design devices

**Table 1.** Some programmable features of modern pacemakers

| |
|---|
| Control and pacing parameters |
| External trigger capability for both chambers |
| Transmission of operating data (e.g., battery voltage, electrode resistance, self-test results) |
| Testing of pacing thresholds |
| Storage of patient data |
| Acquisition, real-time transmission, processing and storage of physiological data |
| Acquisition and processing of data from physiological sensors (temperature, acid-base, transthoracic impedance, QT interval, etc.) |

that offered atrial and ventricular (dual-chamber) demand pacing combined with P-wave triggered ventricular pacing (DDD).

Today, most advanced pacemakers combine DDD pacing with other features that greatly expand indications for the device, as well as facilitate postoperative management of the patient and patient follow-up. Noninvasive two-way communication between the implanted pacemaker and an external programmer provides access to programmable features (Table 1).

Despite the increase in complexity of pacemaker technology, today's devices are smaller, more reliable, and offer an increased service time compared to earlier devices [22]. In the sections which follow, the technological and physiological aspects of artificial pacing, as well as the current state of development, will be examined and illustrated. This assessment will be supplemented with an overview toward the next generation of pacemakers.

## Multiprogrammable Single-Chamber Pacemaker

The use of single-chamber pacemakers prevails in antibradycardiac pacing. Depending on the indication, they are used for pacing either the atrium (AAI, M) or the ventricle (VVI, M). Multiprogrammability, denoted by "M" following the generic pacing codes, permits the adaptation of the implant to a form of electrotherapy that is optimized for each patient. Multiprogrammability offers the advantage of postoperative, noninvasive adjustment of pacing therapy. In addition, it effectively reduces the multiplicity of pacemaker types, a distinct, economic advantage. Table 2 summarizes the programmable parameters for single-chamber pacemakers and their therapeutic and diagnostic significance.

Expanding on Table 2, programmability of the pacing impulse parameters not only overcomes ineffective pacing (e.g., with increased pacing thresholds), but also achieves effective energy savings permitting an extension of useful service time. By providing for noninvasive adjustment of the sensitivity of the cardiac signal detection channels and the possibility to select between a unipolar and bipolar electrode configuration, protection is provided against detection of extraneous (internal, external) signals. Programming of rate and refractory periods is useful for optimizing pacing parameters to the requirements of therapy. Lower-limit rate programming also favors the patient's own heart rhythm if only an occasional need for pacing exists. Finally, a hysteresis setting serves to avoid interference between artificial pacing and an intrinsic rhythm when the two rates are nearly the same [23].

## Technical Solution for the Multiprogrammable Single-Chamber Pacemaker

The block circuit diagram (Figure 2) provides an overall view of the operational principle of a modern, multiprogrammable single-chamber pacemaker. The sensing and output amplifiers of the pacemakers are connected to the myocardium through the electrode. Impulse output energy is adjusted via the amplitude and duration of the pacing pulse. Like the sensitivity of the input amplifier, these variables are controlled

**Table 2.** Clinical significance of programmable parameters for multiprogrammable single-chamber pacemakers.

| Parameter | Diagnostic benefit | Therapeutic benefit |
|---|---|---|
| Rate | Arrhythmia analysis, cardiac output studies, evaluation of competitive rhythms | Optimal pacing rate, overdrive pacing |
| Pulse energy (pulse duration, pulse amplitude) | Threshold analysis safety margin, testing for possible syncope or dizzy spells, temporary suppression of pacing pulses for ECG morphology | Minimizing output energy, prevention of phrenic nerve stimulation, prolongation of service life |
| High pulse energy | Electrode performance | Regaining of capture when threshold has increased, reduction of the number of revisions, prevention of post-operative exit blocks due to acute threshold rises, available reserve energy for electrode instability |
| Sensitivity | Electrode performance, noise evaluation | Correction of entrance block, prevention of oversensing (myopotentials, electromagnetic interference) |
| Hysteresis[a] | Arrhythmia analysis | Provide priority for sinus rhythm |
| Refractory period | Analysis of control dysfunctions | Prevention of T-wave and polarization potential sensing |
| Pacing modes | Hemodynamic evaluation of different modes | Pacing modes adapted to patient's needs |

[a]Amount (time) by which pacemaker escape interval exceeds the pacemaker automatic (pacing) interval.

digitally from the program memory. The central, crystal oscillator-controlled timer and counter are used for the time sequencing of all control processes, such as pacing rate, refractory period, hysteresis, and data transfer. Bidirectional inductive telemetry is used to exchange data with the implant by means of an external programming unit. Programming takes place via a coil, a receiving amplifier, a decoder, a controller, and register in which the temporary and permanent programs are stored. An encoder and a program output stage make available the actual pacing and control parameters, operating parameters (battery current, battery voltage, internal battery resistance, electrode resistance, patient information, etc.), as well as intracardiac electrogram signals and markers [24].

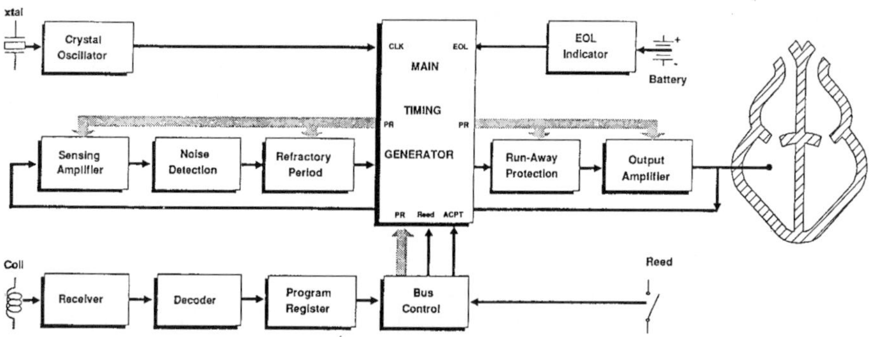


**Fig. 2.** Modern multiprogrammable, single-chamber pacemaker. *EOL,* end of life

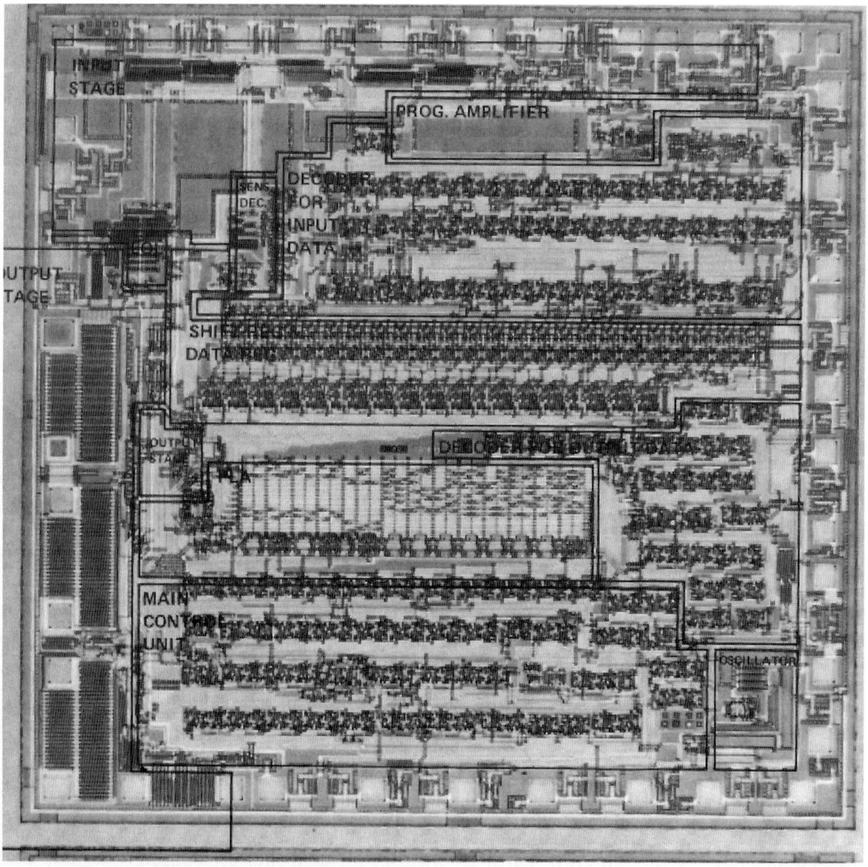


**Fig. 3.** Integrated circuits on silicon chip for monolithic design of single-chamber pacemaker

An example of such a multiprogrammable pacemaker developed using complementary metal oxide semiconductor (CMOS) technology is the monolithic design shown in Fig. 3. All analog and digital functions are integrated on a silicon chip 4 mm x 4 mm in size. The control signals are amplified in a two-stage, band-pass amplifier with eight sensitivity ranges. The pace impulse amplitude is generated by means of a voltage multiplier and can be adjusted between 2.4 and 9.6 V. The topographic arrangement shows the position of the signal, program and output amplifiers, as well as the position of the memory, the oscillator, the reference voltage, the various digital components, and the programmable logic array (PLA); 3-μm silicon gate technology is used. On an area of 16 $mm^2$, about 5000 gates and transistors perform the pacemaker functions. When inhibited, the circuit consumes 5 μA operating current. Under a standard program with a pacing rate of 70 $min^{-1}$ and an output voltage of 4.8 V, the circuit consumes about 15 μA.

Figure 4 shows the assembled pacemaker unit. Hybrid technology is used to establish the connection between the monolithic circuit (Figure 3) and the passive components of the pacemaker electronics [25, 26]. The hybrid is manufactured using thick-film technology. The integrated circuit is hermetically encapsulated in a chip carrier. A coil situated under the hybrid substrate is used for bidirectional telemetry. The lithium battery is located in the left part of the housing. The pacemaker housing consists of a two-part titanium capsule, which is long-term corrosion proof and is hermetically sealed by means of laser- or electron-beam welding. The cast epoxy-

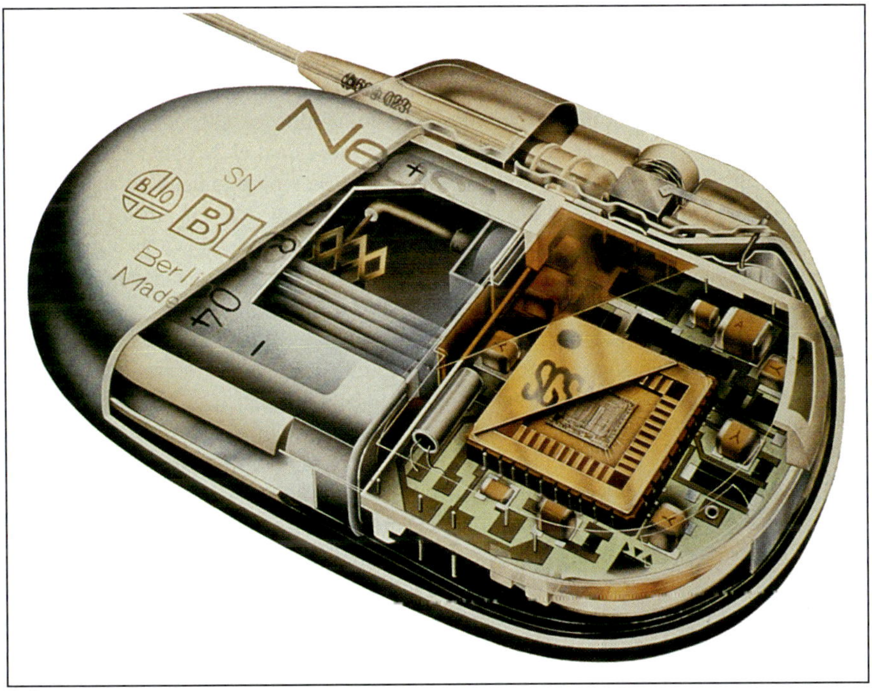

**Fig. 4.** Assembled unit of a modern, multiprogrammable, single-chamber pacemaker

resin head with a connecting block and a vacuum feedthrough forms the electrode connection block.

The high quality of these monolithic circuits and their hybrid structure has been clinically proven in more than 200,000 implants. Reliability of $= 10^{-7}\ h^{-1}$ with a confidence level of 90% for the hybridized overall circuit and $= 10^{-9}\ h^{-1}$ for integrated circuits and passive components has been achieved [27]. In pacemaker technology, reliability cannot be achieved by the usual methods of redundancy of critical circuits and components, since this would entail an increased power consumption. Due to the volume limitations on battery capacity, the requirements for the operating time can only be met if the circuit exhibits a low-power consumption. The quality requirements can only be met by a high degree of integration, good design practices, and the consistent application of control measures in the various phases of manufacture. The latter includes a 100% final testing of the components, semi-finished goods, and the finished product.

## Multiprogrammable Dual-Chamber Pacemaker

With intact SA impulse formation and conduction, but in the presence of AV conduction disturbances, electronic bridging of the AV block through P-wave-controlled pacing of the ventricles (VAT) is the obvious choice. Abnormal atrial excitation, as with premature supraventricular beats or retrogradely conducted ventricular extrasystoles or rhythms, severely restrict the broad application of VAT pacing. Consequently, dual-chamber pacemaker with atrial and ventricular control circuits have been developed (DDD). These devices provide physiological pacing of the atria and ventricles with nearly all possible cardiac rhythm disturbances.

As with a single-chamber unit, multiprogrammability of all control and pacing parameters allows adaptation of the pacemaker to individual electrophysiological and hemodynamic requirements, as well as facilitates the management of the patient throughout the service time of the device. In a universal dual-chamber pacemaker (DDD), atrial or ventricular pacing and control can be selectively switched off. Thus, this pacemaker allows the programmability of all known single- and dual-chamber pacing modes as well as many other features (Table 3) [28].

With a DDD pacemaker, the ventricles are artificially synchronized with the atria by technical means, analogous to the natural excitation sequence. Sensing and pacing are time synchronized with atrial depolarization [29]. AV delay, as well as the atrial and ventricular refractory periods, control the pacing sequence. Automatic adaptation of AV delay to heart rate permits optimization of the hemodynamic contribution of the atrium toward filling the ventricle. The same is true for shortening of the AV delay after a detected P-wave (AV delay fallback), provided to compensate for the latency time between the atrial pulse and its response. Finally, the occurence of pacemaker-mediated arrhythmias or tachycardias as the consequence of ventricular extrasystoles, which are conducted retrogradely to the atria can be prevented by selecting suitable control (refractory) periods.

**Table 3.** Clinical significance of programmable parameters for a multiprogrammable dual-chamber pacemaker

| Parameter | Diagnostic benefit | Therapeutic benefit |
|---|---|---|
| Polarity (pacing and sensing) | ECG recognition of pacing pulses | Elimination of muscle twitching; improving signal-to-noise ratio |
| Dynamic AV delay | Hemodynamic and electrophysiological studies | Improving exercise tolerance; prevention of PMT and reentry SVT |
| Pacing modes DDD with and without dual demand modality | Hemodynamic studies | Maintaining hemodynamic benefits of DDD mode even in the presence of intermittent atrial arrhythmias |
| Pacing mode DDI | Hemodynamic studies | Maintaining AV synchrony in the absence of spontaneous rhythm, no triggering of ventricular pulses by atrial activity |
| Pacing mode DDD with AVT modality | Electrophysiological studies | Prevention of supraventricular reentry tachycardias |
| Pacing modes AAT, VVT, DDT and DDI/T | Sensing tests, chest wall stimulation for series drug testing and for hemodynamic studies | Chest wall stimulation for acute therapy of tachyarrhythmias |
| External pulse triggering by coded signals | Pulse triggering independent of pacemaker timing cycles for electrophysiological studies | Acute therapy of tachyarrhythmias |
| Temporary programming | Test programs for follow-up | Optimization of pacemaker therapy |
| Measurement of battery and lead parameters | Information on current consumption and remaining service time; functional analysis of pacing system; electrode performance studies | Optimization of pacemaker therapy |
| Event counter/ rate histogram | Testing for effectiveness of drug therapy; analysis of long-term performance of pacing systems | Adaptation of drug therapy; optimization of pacemaker therapy |
| Automatic IEGM storage | Arrhythmia analysis; analysis of long-term performance of pacing system | |
| IEGM transmission with marker signals | Arrhythmia analysis; pacing system analysis; interpretation pacemaker ECGs | |

SVT, supraventricular tachycardia; PMT, pacemaker-mediated tachycardia; IEGM, intracardiac electrogram

## Technical Solution for the Dual-Chamber Pacemaker

Similar to the single-chamber pacemaker, the universal DDD pacemaker consists of analog and digital subassemblies. The main structural difference is that the multiprogrammable dual-chamber pacemaker requires two parallel channels for processing of the intracardiac EGMs and for pacing (Fig. 5), and the hybrid circuit for such a

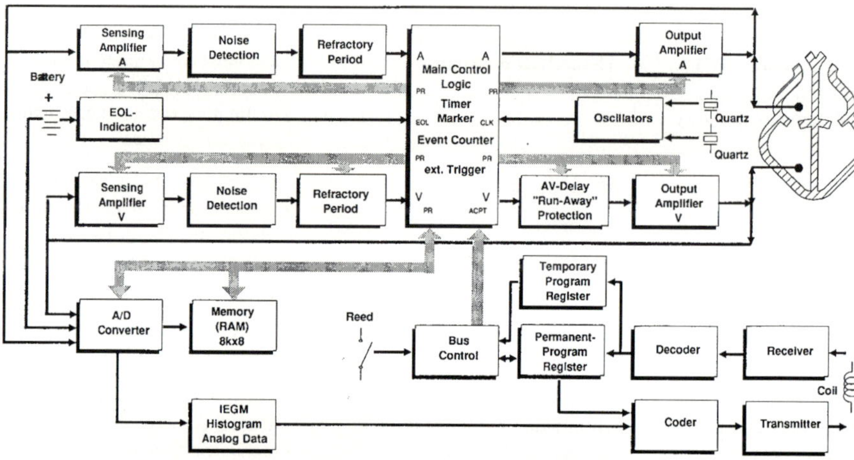


**Fig.5.** Multiprogrammable, dual-chamber pacemaker (DDDM) permitting intracardiac electrogram analysis and containing patient data memory. *EOL,* end of life; *PR,* P or R potential; *CLK,* clock; *ACPT,* accepted

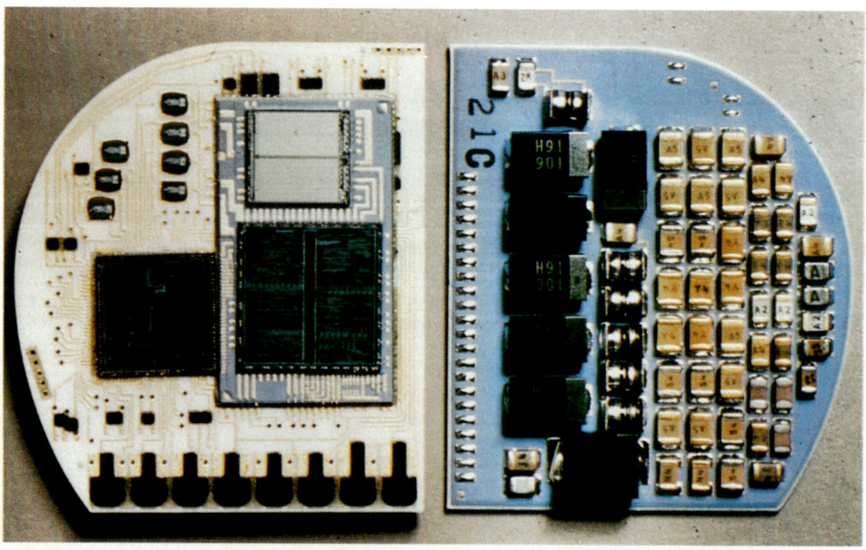

**Fig. 6.** Hybrid circuit for multiprogrammable, dual-chamber pacemaker, front and back sides

pacemaker in Fig. 6. The multistage bandpass amplifiers for the acquisition of the intracardiac atrial and ventricular signals, together with the analog data processing circuits, the voltage multiplier, the output stage, and the telemetry unit are collected together on one integrated circuit. The digital signal processing and control unit is likewise designed monolithically. In conjunction with the separate memory chip (RAM), it forms the central logic and data acquisition unit. The capacitors and the input protection diodes are assembled on the back side of the hybrid circuit. The technical task of reestablishing the natural excitation process consists of synchronizing the ventricles with the atria. The control logic circuitry evaluates signals from the atrium and the ventricle and secures pacing in accordance with need [30]. In the dual-chamber mode, the states "sensed" and "paced" can be formally defined for both chambers, so that four basic states with their transitions can be distinguished: atrium sensed, atrium paced, ventricle sensed, ventricle paced.

State sequencing is performed by a control unit (controller). The essential components of the controller are the state register and the random logic block. The state register stores the current status of the system and also conveys this information to the logic block. The logic block, depending on the current state and other input signals, operates a collection of programmable timers (timer file). The latter, if necessary, will change the pacemaker's state with the next cycle of the system time clock. Additionally, the logic block generates signals for the output register, which controls the analog circuit parts in accordance with its programmed instructions. Finally, various execution sequences of the state register are selected through a mode-control register. Thus, in the DDD mode of operation a multiprogrammable pacemaker controller executes the four basic states (as mentioned above) with a number of possible transitions and generates several pacemaker timing intervals and refractory or blanking periods (Fig. 7).

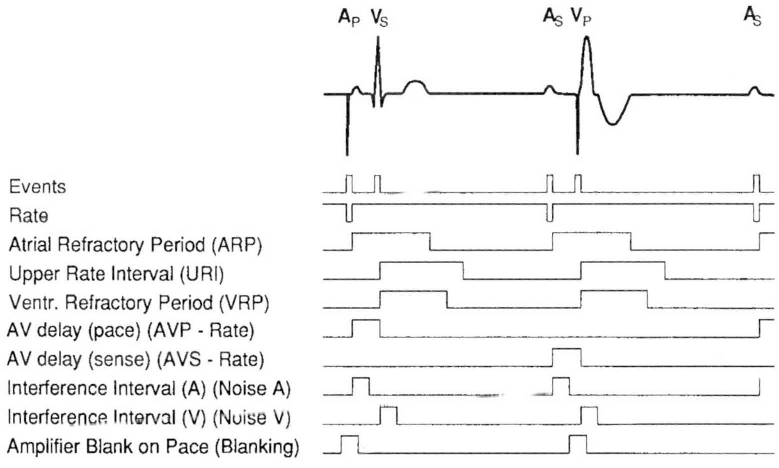


**Fig. 7.** Correlation between ECG signals and pacemaker timing intervals or refractory periods for multiprogrammable, dual-chamber pacemaker

The control unit also offers rhythm monitoring through internal analysis and transmission of intracardiac electrograms. Arrhythmias are analyzed in real time, and up to three atrial and ventricular electrograms can be stored and processed. Several event counters are provided to monitor the pacing and sensing activity and are used for arrhythmia diagnosis. The pacemaker can also be used for electrophysiological measurements when linked with appropriate external programming and stimulating units.

## Controlled and Regulated Pacemakers

The multiprogrammable pacemakers discussed have provided patients with improved cardiac function by correcting bradycardic dysrhythmias and restoring proper AV synchrony within the heart. However, in the presence of insufficient chronotropic response to exercise the benefits provided the patient are limited [31]. The only remaining way the regulatory system can adjust cardiac output is through changes in stroke volume (contractility). These changes are limited to approximately 30% – 50% of resting levels. In contrast, changes in heart rate can be expected to increase cardiac output by up to 300%.

To provide patients with a greater cardiovascular adaptation, pacemakers have been designed to be rate-responsive. To various degrees, rate-responsive pacemakers permit workload-dependent adaptation of the pacing rate. Active patients with sinus node dysfunction benefit most from rate-responsive pacemakers. The rate-responsive

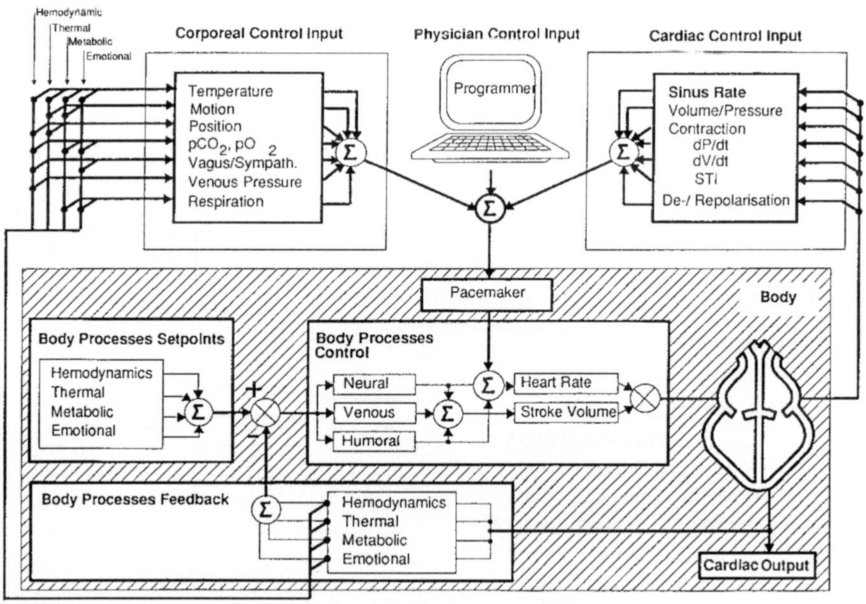


**Fig. 8.** Different body and cardiac control inputs in a general model for rate-adaptive pacing which reestablishes chronotropic control of the heart.

pacemaker system must work with the cardiovascular regulatory processes. Rate-responsive pacemakers mimic the heart's response to cardiovascular regulatory control mechanisms (Fig. 8) [32, 33].

## Status of the Application of Corporeal Control Parameters

Rate-adaptive pacemakers using one or more of the corporeal control input signals (Fig. 8) have been developed. The realization of a rate-adaptive pacemaker based on a sensor signal requires the availability of a suitable transducer and a suitably robust algorithm. Table 4 summarizes the available sensor technology necessary to implement one of these rate-adaptive strategies. The same high-quality requirements imposed on permanent pacemakers also apply to rate-adaptive sensor technology. A stable and reliable measurement function must be maintained for many years. The sensor must be very small and use very little power. As discussed below, there are numerous transducers which meet these requirements and may be incorporated into a rate-adaptive pacemaker [34].

## Motion Energy as a Corporeal Control Parameter

Thoracic motion is sensed by some rate-adaptive pacemakers. A number of refinements to sensing have been made, including improving the sensor to better detect motion associated with physical work and adjustments to the algorithm to better

**Table 4.** Control parameters and sensors for rate-adaptive pacemakers

| Control parameter | Sensor | Evaluation |
|---|---|---|
| P-wave parameter | Atrial lead | Ideal control |
| Respiration parameter | Intrathoracic impedance | Open loop |
| QT-time parameter | Stimulation electrode | Open loop |
| Activity control | Piezoelectric sensor | Nonmetabolic parameter |
| $O_2$saturation | Optical transducer | Open loop parameter |
| Blood temperature | Thermistor electrode | Semi-closed loop parameter |
| PEP control | Unipolar impedance electrode | Closed loop |
| Stroke volume control | Multipolar impedance elcctrode | Closed loop |

PEP, preejection period

discriminate between valid and invalid signals [35, 36]. An important improvement was to shift the sensor from a frequency detector to an energy detector, when it was determined that a direct relationship exists between motion energy and heart rate. In many forms of exercise, the activity of large muscle groups is the most important component of total body work and oxygen consumption. Measurements of the relative motions of the body mass, therefore, suffices as an estimate of whole body ergometry [37–39].

The following correlations provide the basis for a motion-energy, rate-adaptive pacemaker. Body motion is correlated with large muscle activity, which in terms correlates with muscle $O_2$ consumption. Increases in the latter must be supported by an increased cardiac output. To provide the latter, the sensor-driven pacing rate is increased. The effectiveness of the motion-energy, rate-adaptive pacemaker rests on the strength and selectivity of these correlations [40, 41]. The strength of the correlation is also dependent on signal detection, signal processing, and the control algorithm. These constraints apply equally well to all corporeal control variables which more or less correlate with actual cardiac demand [42].

A mechanism for monitoring motion energy is required. The physical laws of mechanics, i.e., conservation of energy and momentum, are applicable. The sensor must detect and quantify motion or acceleration. Placing the motion sensor in the pacemaker can allow it to detect motions with the largest expenditures of energy. Pacemaker acceleration or thoracic tissue vibrations can be detected and used as indicators of energy expenditure. The sensor must be very stable and exhibit low power dissipation. The piezoelectric sensor meets these criteria: it is very stable and does not require an external power source and has been used in sports medicine for ergometry for some time [35].

In designing a sensor circuit, one must consider that the measurement signal is dominated by frequencies below the resonance frequency of the piezoelectric transducer. Therefore, measurements must be proportional to the acceleration, and signals are integrated by a seven-stage circuit to obtain signals which are proportional to the motion energy. The design of the sensor and integrator circuitry is applicable to both single- and dual-chamber pacemakers. Further, the combination of P-wave sensing (Table 4) with body motion detection offers the advantage of an even broader range of therapeutic strategies.

A rate-adaptive pacemaker must provide additional programmable features to tailor device performance to the patient's clinical requirements. Useful programmable features are sensor sensitivity, maximum pacing rates and response times. Programming the sensor sensitivity allows parameter adjustment to the unique biomechanical and anatomical characteristics of the patient. Maximum pacing rate programming permits prescription of a pacing range consistent with the patient's medical history and cardiac reserves. Programming response times will determine how rapidly the pacing rate is to increase with the onset of physical activity and how slowly it will return to the resting rate upon cessation of physical activity. Response times can be adjusted to keep the patient free of symptoms during the transition period between resting and active states.

Programmable sensor sensitivity along with response times permit adaptation of therapeutic pacing rates to low workloads. Thus, the sensor-controlled pacemaker can

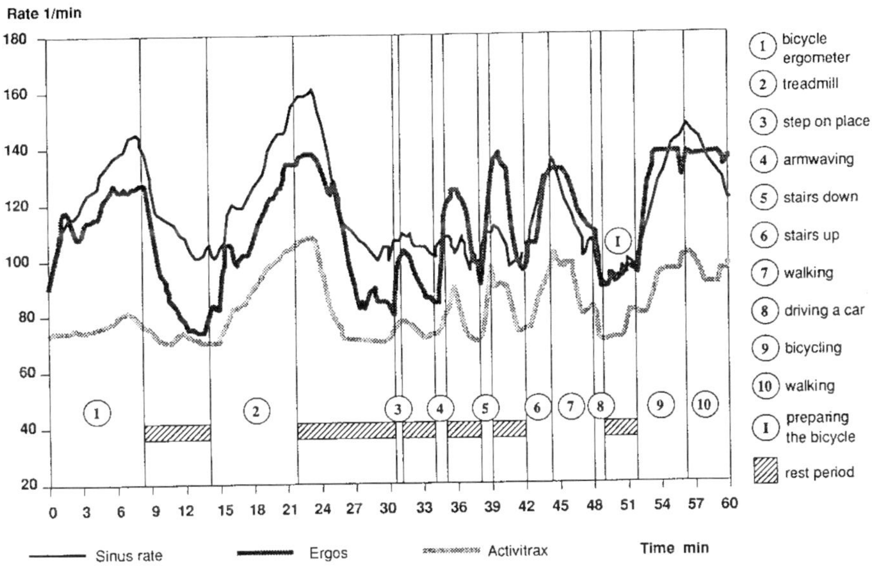


**Fig. 9.** Comparison of sinus rate response during exercise with rates achieved by two types of motion-sensor pacemakers: motion-energy sensing (Ergos) vs. motion-frequency sensing (Activitrax)

be made to respond when the patient sits up or stands up. Such rapid response behavior is particularly valuable for patients with orthostatic circulatory insufficiency.

While the motion-energy, rate-adaptive pacemaker is effective in providing a pacing rate responsive to the patient's needs under a wide range of conditions, motion energy is not the only algorithm which might be used in conjuction with a piezoelectric accelerometer. Motion frequency may also be used. In the case of the motion-frequency algorithm, the pacing rate is controlled by the frequency with which the sensor signal exceeds some preselected threshold value. The frequency-based algorithm, however, does not perform well in normal daily activities such as climbing stairs or hills. For example, when ascending stairs, elderly patients typically decrease their stepping cadence, while at the same time increasing their level exertion. Under these conditions, the frequency-based algorithm inappropriately decreases pacing rate. Figure 9 depicts results of a comparative study where two types of motion-sensor pacemakers were externally attached to the thorax of test subjects. Note that the pacing control algorithm based on motion energy exhibits better specification than one based on motion frequency. Further, the rate response of the motion-energy device more nearly approximates the sinus rate response [43].

## Central Venous Temperature as Corporeal Control Parameter

The application of the central venous temperature (CVT) to the control of the pacing frequency is based on the work of Csapo's group [44]. As confirmed by later studies a

**Table 5.** Advantages of central venous temperatures as a control parameter for rate-adaptive pacing

| |
|---|
| Physiological adaptation of paced rate to meet individual patient needs with physical stress |
| Sensing of circadian variations in temperature permits physiological adaptation of paced rate during sleep |
| Physiological adaptation of paced rate in response to fever and other hypermetabolic states |
| Rapid adaptation of paced rate in response to high workloads (> 50 W) |

linear relationship exists between the CVT, the workload, and the chronotropic heart rate [44, 45]. Multistage averaging permits a differentiation between workload-independent (circadian) and workload-dependent temperature fluctuations. In this way, both types of temperature fluctuations can be used for physiological rate adaptation to metabolic needs, especially during sleep at night [45, 46, 47, 48]. A rapid rise in pacing rate at the beginning of exercise can be achieved by referring the workload-specific temperature rise to a continually updated reference value, which reflects the workload-independent, slow temperature variations [49, 50].

The technical solution for temperature-sensing, rate-adaptive pacing makes use of a single chip microcomputer that includes a microprocessor, timer and counter functions, system read/write memory (RAM, 112 byte), and program memory (ROM, 2 kbyte). An external data memory (RAM, 8 kbyte x 8) is used to store all programmed control parameters and to manage patient and diagnostic measurement data. These are especially important since, after being interrogated via the programming unit, they permit rapid adjusting and setting of the parameters that are essential for rate control. For example, a record of the temperature behavior over a 24-h period can be documented graphically. These diagnostic data can be programmed into the pacemaker by an external programming unit and therefore made available for optimal adjustment of the implanted unit. The system temperature acquisition unit consists of a thermistor (integrated into the pacing electrode) and an analog-integrated circuit with a digital interface for temperature measurement (resolution ± 0.025°C). Pacemaker functions are provided by a separate integrated circuit.

Clinical experience confirms the workload specification of CVT for controlled rate adaptation [51–56]. Temperature-controlled rate adaptation appears physiologically for all workload stages. Based on metabolic relationship, the advantages of CVT as a control for rate-adaptive pacing are listed in Table 5.

## Cardiac Control Parameters

Rate-adaptive pacemakers responsive to cardiac signals have been developed. The realization of such pacemakers requires detection of suitable signals and availability of practical algorithms. Table 4 lists sensors used to implement a cardiac control strategy. In comparison to corporeal control parameters, cardiac control parameters offer the general advantage that the sensed cardiac variable already contains systemic control information (e.g., neural input) [32]. Cardiac parameters which contain neural and other control information include SA rate, ventricular stroke volume, systolic time intervals, and the QT interval of the ECG. To work in conjunction with the autonomic cardiovascular regulatory system, the ideal sensed cardiac control signal should be proportional to sympathetic tone and independent of heart rate [55, 56].

The latter condition is not strictly satisfied by the QT time interval [57]. The QT interval shortens not only with an increase in sympathetic tone but also with increased heart rate. Consequently, to avoid possible rate instability with positive feedback conditions, a useful QT interval control algorithm must account for dependence of the QT interval on both neural input and heart rate.

### Preejection Period as Cardiac Control Variable

The Preejection Period (PEP) is one example of a systolic time interval which contains sympathetic control information. PEP is defined as the time from the beginning of the depolarization of the ventricles to the opening of the aortic valve. PEP, therefore, includes a number of phases of the cardiac cycle. Contraction begins after a slight delay for electrical excitation and depolarization. This interval is called the electromechanical lag. It is followed by the isovolumetric contraction phase of the cardiac cycle. During this phase the ventricular pressure rises rapidly while the valves remain closed and the ventricular volume remains constant. The ejection phase begins at the end of this process with opening of the aortic and pulmonary valves [58–60].
At fixed spontaneous or paced heart rates, cardiac output can only be increased by an increase in stroke volume, achieved via the Frank-Starling mechanism, or an increase in contractility mediated by sympathetic stimulation. These factors lead to an increase in the force and speed of contraction. The more rapid pressure rise in the ventricles shortens the time until the pulmonary or aortic valves open. Thus, PEP is inversely proportional to the inotropic state of the heart and sympathetic tone [61–63].

The PEP measured in the right ventricle (RV-PEP) shows the same behavior as that in the left ventricle (LV-PEP). RV-PEP, therefore, is also a useful indicator of the contractile state of the heart. There exists a direct relationship between myocardial contractility and the normal pulse rate. Exploitation of this relationship provides a rate-adaptive pacing control parameter with high sensitivity and specification, so that PEP is now used as an input signal for rate-adaptive pacemakers [64–68].

### Cardiac Impedance Measurements

Analogous to plethysmographic impedance measurements, the cardiac impedance may be recorded using a unipolar pacing lead in the right ventricle (Fig. 10) [69–76]. The point of impedance change associated with the end of the isovolumetric contraction phase and the beginning of the rapid ejection phase of the cardiac cycle can be identified (circles on the Z recording). The corresponding point of maximum negative impedance slope (dZ/dt) is a reliable end point for determining PEP [77, 78]. Cardiac

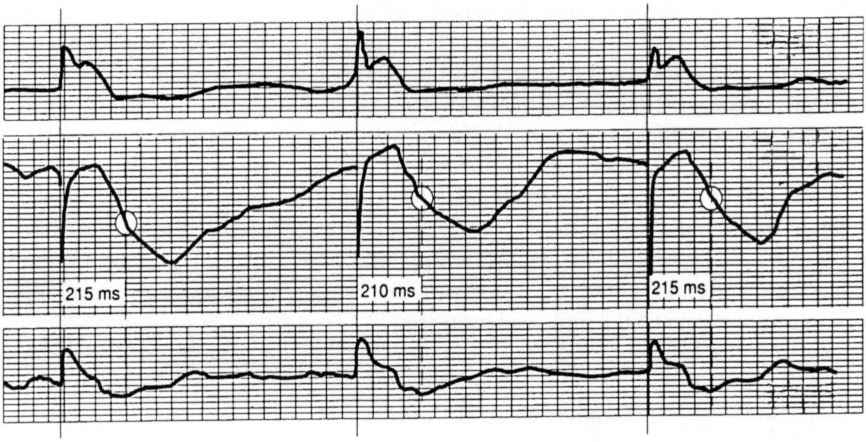


**Fig. 10.** Simultaneous recordings of right ventricular electrogram (ECG, *top*), impedance (Z, middle) and dZ/dt (*bottom*)

impedance is measured by injecting alternating current (I = 40 μA, F = 4 KHz, square wave) into the pacing electrode. This current is more than an order of magnitude below the stimulation threshold, but large enough to reliably detect small impedance variations associated with ventricular systole. Expected values for impedance are several hundred ohms, with systolic changes in impedance ranging from 5 to 30 ohms. The current-induced voltage is measured at 8 msec intervals with a 4 ms sampling period. The 4 msec sampling period corresponds to 16 pulses of the supplied excitation (alternating) current. The impedance signal is measured with a bandwidth of about 40 Hz. The useful signal change during the contraction phase amounts to a maximum of 1 mV. During the measurement portion of the cardiac cycle, other digital activities are kept to a minimum to reduce electrical interference.

After amplification and filtering, the impedance signal is detected by means of a synchronous demodulator as a DC voltage proportional to the impedance change. Compared to simple rectification, synchronous demodulation offers the advantage that high frequency noise is not demodulated into the signal band or can be readily suppressed by subsequent filters. After demodulation, the impedance signal is processed by a bandpass filter and a programmable gain amplifier stage which can be adjusted in eight steps. After further amplification and filtering, the signal is fed into an A/D converter. At the end of the measurement time, the converter makes the impedance signal available to the digital signal processing system.

To minimize the pacemaker operating current, impedance measurements are restricted to that portion of the cardiac cycle during which the end of PEP is expected to occur. This is permissible since circulatory regulatory processes occur relatively slowly. Thus, the measurement window can be kept narrow and positioned relative to the most recently determined PEP value. If temporary interference prevents PEP determinations, a larger window size is set automatically.

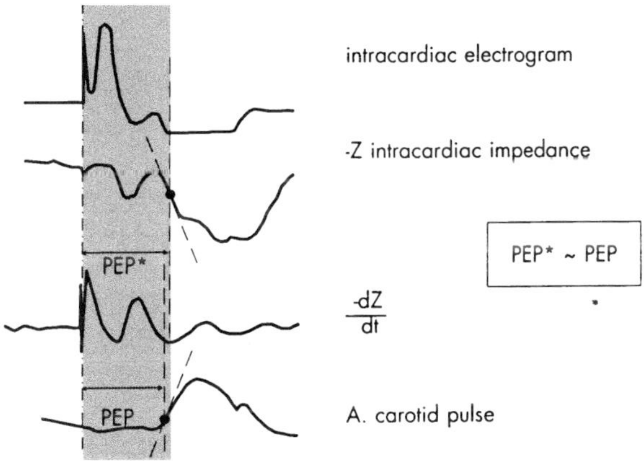


**Fig. 11.** Determination of PEP using right ventricular impedance curve (PEP*). Note that PEP* determined this way is nearly the same as PEP determined from the carotid wave form

With a maximum measurement window size of 256 ms, 32 measurements are made per cardiac cycle. Fluctuations in the impedance signal are further reduced using a two-dimensional digital filter. One dimension of the filter acts in the cardiac cycle time domain. The other filter acts on corresponding points of successive cardiac cycles. The resulting impedance wave form is used to determine the PEP end point (Fig. 11). The derivate of the filtered impedance wave form is calculated to identify the time of occurrence of the maximum slope. This time point is defined as the PEP value for the current cardiac cycle. The programmed heart rate is assigned to the PEP value by way of a formula or table. The PEP-to-pacing rate transfer functions can be quite complex. In the simplest case, it follows the equation [63]:

$$HR = \frac{6 \cdot 10^5}{K_2\,(PEP\text{-}K_1)}$$

Transfer functions are stored as programmable tables in the pacemaker. The tables allow for maximum flexibility in defining the transfer functions. Redundant software and hardware measures are used to prevent run away pacing rates in the event of hardware or software errors. A reduction in the number of impedance measurements per cardiac cycle reduces power consumption. Provision of a dynamic search window (sliding window) further reduces power consumption. Energy is conserved by suppressing impedance measurements at times of prolonged patient inactivity. Finally, dialogue with an external programming unit is carried on in two ways. When the PEP function is switched off, the system behaves like a normal single-chamber, multiprogrammable pacemaker. When the PEP control is on, the PEP-related functions are initiated by the programming unit: (a) recording impedance data; (b) interrogating impedance data; (c) reading and writing patient data; (d) reading event counters, status bits, error bits; (e) writing and reading the PEP parameters.

When used to control pacing rate, PEP is defined as the time between the R-wave or pacing stimulus and the maximum negative slope of the intraventricular impedance curve (Fig. 11). That PEP is inversely proportional to the intrinsic (sinus) heart rate. Measured PEP and sinus or calculated heart rates during rest, exercise, and recovery from exercise are shown for one subject in Fig. 12. However, if the heart rate changes

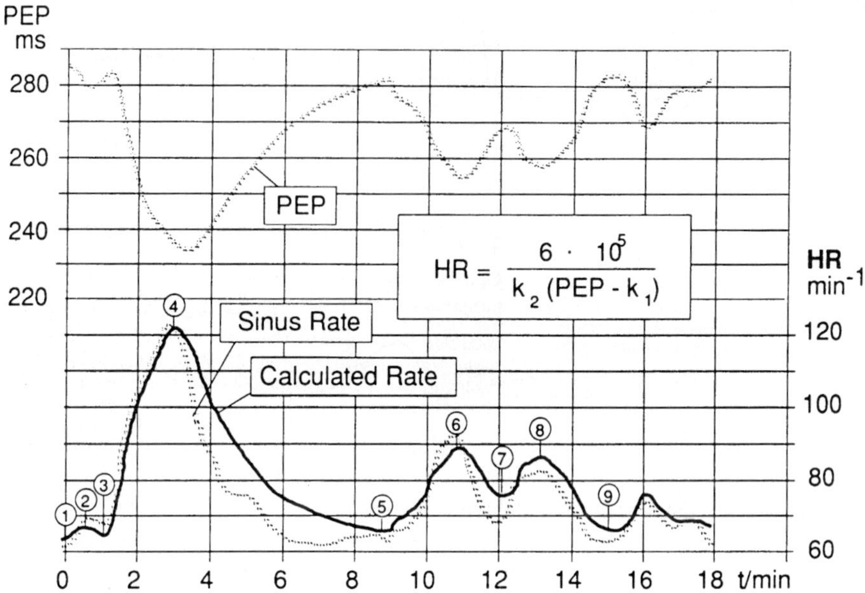


**Fig. 12.** Measured PEP and sinus or calculated heart rates for one subject during rest, exercise, and recovery from exercise. *1,* Rest; *2,* speaking; *3,* exercise; *4,* recovery (sitting); *5,* climbing stairs; *6,* recovery (sitting); *7,* going downstairs; *8,* recovery (sitting); *9,* going to next room

without an adrenergic influence, e.g., by artificial pacing while at a constant cardiac demand, PEP remains constant.

## Rate-Adaptive Pacing Controlled by Cardiac Impedance-Based PEP Measurements

The principle of a pacemaker which is rate-controlled by means of right ventricular PEP based on cardiac impedance measurements has attained clinical significance. Fig. 13 shows the typical regulation behavior of the PEP-controlled pacemaker. Under exercise stress, PEP is shortened with the decrease in PEP and increase in calculated heart rate exhibiting a nearly linear relationship. The software of this particular pacemaker accounted for possible changes in ventricular preload with changes in posture. The reliability of using PEP as a control parameter is evident from Fig. 13. Further, the concept is relatively simple and has the distinct clinical advantage of using standard pacemaker electrodes both for pacing and for PEP measurements. Because of its dependence on sympathetic tone, PEP is a reliable parameter for adapting the heart rate to changes in physical workload. Rate-adaptation is fast, relatively trouble free, physiological, and prevents stressing the contractile reserve of the heart unnecessarily. Thus, PEP-controlled, rate-adaptive pacemakers hold out the promise of more closely modeling natural regulatory control of the heart.

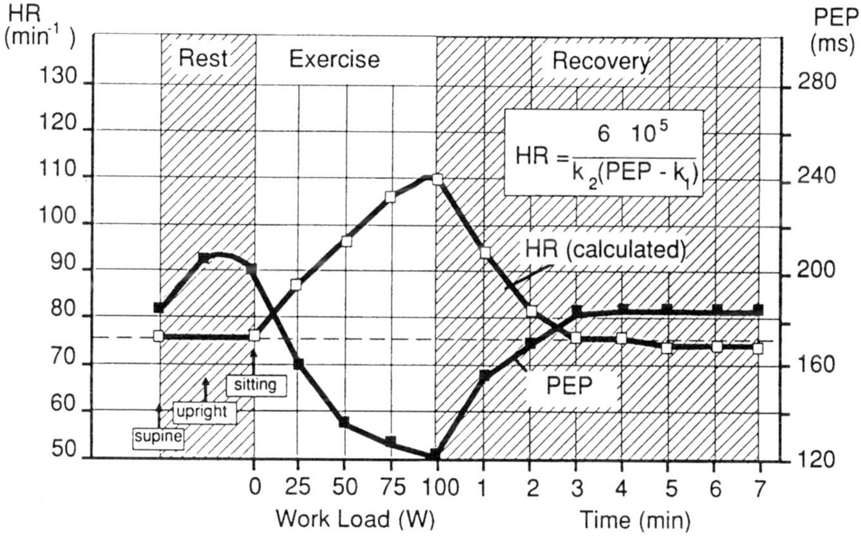


**Fig. 13.** Typical regulation behavior for rate-adaptive pacemaker controlled by cardiac impedance-based PEP measurements. *HR*, heart rate

## Volume Control

To increase cardiac output, three mechanisms are available to the heart: (1) augmentation of end-diastolic volume (preload) as the result of increased venous return, (2) reduction of end-systolic volume caused by increased contractility, and (3) an increase in heart rate.

In healthy individuals with normal ventricular loading conditions, only the last two of these mechanisms can be observed. Augmentation of preload, however, becomes important if the heart rate is low compared to the workload level. Thus, within certain limits, the heart can adapt to match the actual requirements, even if heart rate remains constant. The same is true for artificially introduced rate changes with constant workloads, so that the stroke volume will adjust opposite to rate changes to keep cardiac output at or close to the level necessary to satisfy metabolic needs.

This negative feedback relation between heart rate and stroke volume can be used to adapt the rate of an artificial pacemaker [78]. Using this principle, heart rate is controlled by a closed-loop system (Fig. 14). End-diastolic volume or stroke volume represents the regulation variable, pacing rate the actuator variable, and changes in cardiac output a disturbance of the regulator. End-diastolic and stroke volumes are measured by intracardiac impedance plethysmography. A four element (multipolar) right ventricular electrode catheter serves for pacing, sensing, and measurements of impedance used to determine right ventricular volume changes [79].

When compared to other control parameters for rate-adaptive pacing, volume control ideally fulfills the clinical requirement for reestablishing physiological conditions. Volume-controlled pacemakers automatically adapt to the existing performance capability of the myocardium. Preliminary clinical results (unpublished

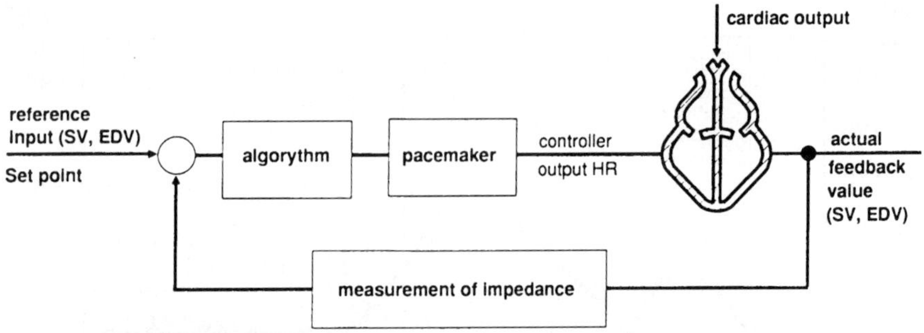


**Fig. 14.** Closed loop control of pacemaker rate by exploiting the negative feedback relation between heart rate (*HR*) and stroke volume (*SV*). *EDV*, end-diastolic volume

observations) confirm that changes in the end-systolic cardiac volume are indicators of a change in CO demand. By adjusting the heart rate to support the change in CO demand, the pacemaker automatically adjusts to the remaining cardiac reserve. In a manner analogous to autonomic regulation of the heart rate, volume-controlled adaptation of the pacing rate has the advantage that the pacing rate tracks along with a rise in cardiac output, within the theoretical range of the stroke volume. Therefore, it optimally models natural circulatory regulation.

## Reestablishment of Physiological Regulation: A Challenge to Technology

The exemplary collaboration in recent decades between the engineering and medical sciences has developed electrotherapy of the heart into an extremely successful therapy. Due to technological advances, cardiac pacemakers can now reliably reestablish cardiovascular function and improve the quality of life in a large group of patients. Their superiority over previous forms of pacing treatment arise from the utilization of remaining physiological adaptation and regulatory processes still available to the cardiovascular system in patients with heart disease. More complete understanding of normal cardiac impulse formation and conduction, and their replacement by artificial processes, have further strengthened success with the aforementioned interdisciplinary efforts.

Microelectronics is a key technology in biomedical data collection and processing in many areas of medical engineering. Permanent implantation of electronic cardiac pacemakers became possible with the introduction of the first electronic components of semiconductor physics. The small number of discrete transistors used in the earliest models of pacemakers have been replaced by complex components which combine thousands of these elements on an area of a few square millimeters. The analog and digital functions of the cardiac pacemaker are now assembled using very large scale integration technology and integrated circuits. Modular elements of such circuits can only be seen under a microscope. Complex electrical functions such as counters and oscillators, charge pumps and memories, analog/digital converters, and microprocessors have been miniaturized to the point where they are now invisible to the naked eye.

The advanced state of the electronic technologies has led to broad clinical applications supporting a wide range of pacing therapies. The classical form of physiological rate-adaptive pacing is dual-chamber sensing and pacing (DDD pacing). With AV heart block, but with intact SA impulse formation and conduction, improved hemodynamic results are obtained when AV synchrony can be included in the pacing process. However, the DDD pacemaker fails if it tracks nonphysiological atrial rates. Modern pacemaker technology has met the challenge by adopting other strategies.

Pacemakers now in clinical trials achieve rate adaption through the direct control of the pacing rate in response to other physiological signals, including metabolic and other physiological indicators. A further refinement in rate-adaptive pacing has been the introduction of devices which function by cooperating with the intrinsic cardiovascular control processes. Such "optimal" rate adaptive pacemaker systems have been developed based on cardiac impedance plethysmography using the stroke volume or systolic time intervals as regulatory signals. Thus, as in other medical disciplines, advances in microelectronic technology have enabled physicians to implement simpler yet more versatile pacing therapies. Moreover, the current and envisioned states of microelectronic technology hold promise for further advances in pacemaker therapy.

## References


1 Antoni H (1985) Funktion des Herzens. In: Schmidt RF, Thews G (eds) Physiologie des Menschen. Springer, Berlin Heidelberg New York, p 391

2 Guyton AC (1968) Textbook of medical physiology, 3 rd edn. Saunders, Philadelphia

3 Schmidt RF, Thews G (1985) Physiologie des Menschen. Springer, Berlin Heidelberg New York

4 Trautwein W (1972) Erregungsphysiologie des Herzens. In: Gauer F, Kramer KG, Jung E (eds) Physiologie des Menschen, vol 3, Urban u. Schwarzenberg, Munich

5 Alt E (1986) Schrittmachertherapie des Herzens. Perimed, Munich

6 Breithardt G, Lüderitz B, Schlepper M (1989) Empfehlungen für die Implantation zur permanenten Schrittmacherimplantation. Z Kardiol 78:212–215

7 Lüderitz B (1986) Herzschrittmacher: Therapie und Diagnostik kardialer Rhythmusstörungen. Springer, Berlin Heidelberg New York, p 430

8 Stangl K, Heuer H, Wirtzfeld A (1990) Frequenzadaptive Herzschrittmacher. Steinkopff, Darmstadt

9 Anderson KM, Moore AA (1986) Sensors in pacing. PACE 9:954–959

10 Camilli L, Alcidi L, Shapland E, Obino S (1983) Results, problems and perspectives with the autoregulating pacemaker. PACE 6:488–493

11 Funke HD (1975) Ein Herzschrittmacher mit belastungsabhängiger Frequenzregulation. Biomed Tech (Berlin) 20:225–228

12 Mehta D, Lau CP, Ward DE, Camm AJ (1988) Comparative evaluation of chronotropic responses of QT-sensing and activity sensing rate responsive pacemaker. PACE 11:1405–1412

13 Nappholz TA, Maloncy JD, Simmons T, Masterson M, Fischer S, Valenta H (1987) A two year research study of minute ventilation as an indicator for rate responsive pacing. PACE 10:1222

14 Schaldach M (1987) Present state and future trends in electrical heart stimulation. Med Prog Technol 13:85–102

15 Stangl K, Wirtzfeld A, Heinze R, Laule M, Seitz K, Göbl G (1988) A new multisensor pacing system using stroke volume, respiratory rate, mixed venous oxygen saturation, and temperature, right atrial pressure, right ventricular pressure, and dP/dt. PACE 11:712–724
16 Wirtzfeld A, Heinze R, Stangl K, Hoekstein K, Alt E, Liess HD (1984) Regulation of pacing rate by variations of mixed venous oxygen saturation. Pace 7:1257–1262
17 Mindt W, Schaldach M (1975) Electrochemical aspects of pacing electrodes. In: Schaldach M, Furman S (eds) Advances in pacemaker technology. Springer, Berlin Heidelberg New York, pp 297–305 (Engineering in medicine, vol 1)
18 Owens J, Boone B (1986) Batteries for implantable biomedical devices. Plenum, New York, pp 358
19 Schaldach M, Hubmann M, Hardt R, Weikl A (1989) Titannitrid-Herzschrittmacher-Elektroden. Biomed Tech (Berlin) 34:185–190
20 Schaldach M, Thull R (1988) Das elektrochemische Verhalten gesinterter Metallelektroden. Biomed Tech (Berlin) 33 (Suppl):333–335
21 Elmquist R, Senning A (1959) Implantable pacemaker for the heart. In: Medical electronics. Proceedings of the 2nd international conference on medical electronics, Paris, June 1959
22 Schaldach M (1987) Reliability considerations in the design of implantable products. Biomed Tech Berlin 32:276–284
23 Friedberg MD, Barold SS (1973) On hysteresis in pacing. J Electrocardiol 6:2
24 Castellanet MJ, Garza J, Shaner SP, Messenger JC (1987) Telemetry of programmed and measured data in pacing system evaluation and follow-up. J Electrophysiol 1:360–375
25 Schaldach M (1990) Die Bedeutung der Mikroelektronik in der Implantattechnologie. Biomed Techn (Berlin) 35 (Suppl 2):3–13
26 Schaldach M (1987) Hybrid microelectronics in implant technology: a progress report. Hybrid Circuit Technol 4:19–26
27 Schaldach M (1986) Stand und Entwicklungstendenzen der Mikroelektronik in der biomedizinischen Technik. Elektronik u. Maschinenbau 103:127–138
28 Bernstein AD, Camm AJ, Fletcher RD, Gold RD, Rickards AF, Smyth NPD, Spielman SR, Sutton R (1987) The NASPE/BPEG generic pacemaker code for antibradyarrhythmia and adaptive-rate pacing and antitachyarrthmia devices. PACE 10:794–799
29 Furman S, Hurzeler P, de Caprio V (1977) The ventricular endocardial electrogram and pacemaker sensing. J Thorac Cardiovasc Surg 73:258–266
30 Schaldach M (1984) Entwicklungstendenzen in der physiologischen Stimulation des Herzens. In: Weikl (ed) Physiologische Stimulation des Herzens. Perimed, Erlangen, pp 134–165
31 Ferrer I (1968) The sick-sinus-syndrome in atrial disease. JAMA 206:645
32 Guyton AC, Coleman TG (1967) Long-term regulation of the circulation: interrelationship with body fluid volumes. In: Reeve EB, Guyton AC (eds) Physical base of circulatory transport: regulation and exchange. Saunders, Philadelphia, pp 179–201
33 Guyton AC, Coleman TG, Granger HJ (1972) Circulation: overall regulation. Ann Rev Physiol 34:13–46
34 Ko WH (1983) A review of implantable sensors. PACE 6:482–487
35 Hubmann M, Weikl A, Hardt R, Schaldach M (1989) Bewegungsenergie als Steuergröße für die Anpassung der Stimulationsfrequenz. Biomed Tech (Berlin) 34:191–196
36 Lau CP, Stott JRR, Toff WD, Zetlein MB, Ward DE, Camm AJ (1988) Selective vibration sensing: a new concept for activity-sensing rate-responsive pacing. PACE 11:1299–1309
37 Reswick J (1978) Preliminary evaluation of the vertical acceleration gait analyzer (VAGA). Proceedings of the 6th annual symposium on the external control of human extremities. Dubrovnik, Yugoslavia, 28. Aug–1. Sept, pp 305–314
38 Servais SB, Webster JG, Montoyo HJ (1978) Estimating human energy expenditure using an accelerometer device. IEEE Front Eng Health Care 309
39 Wong TC, Webster JG, Montoye HJ, Washburn R (1981) Portable accelerometer device for measuring human energy expenditure. IEEE Trans Biomed Eng 28:467–471
40 Humen DP, Anderson K, Brumwell D, Huntley S, Klein GJ (1983) A pacemaker which automatically increases its rate with physical activity. In: Steinbach K (ed) Cardiac pacing. Proceedings of the 7th world symposium on cardiac pacing. Steinkopff, Darmstadt, pp 259–264

41 Humen DP, Kostuk WJ, Klein GJ (1985) Activity sensing rate responsive pacing: improvement in myocardial performance with exercise. PACE 8:52–59
42 Hubmann M, Weikl A, Hardt R, Schaldach M (1989) Frequenzadaptive Herzschrittmacher: Ein Vergleich zwischen impuls- und beschleunigungsproportionaler Steuerung. Biomed Tech (Berlin) 34:57–59
43 Res JCJ, de Boer TJM (1990) Evaluation of a new body motion sensing rate response sensor (Ergos 2), using a multiphase exercise protocol. PACE 13:1207
44 Weisswange A, Csapo G, Perach W, Kannegieber E (1978) Frequenzsteuerung von Schrittmachern durch Bluttemperatur. Verh Dtsch Ges Kreislaufforsch 44:152
45 Aschoff J, Gunther B, Kramer K (1971) Energiehaushalt und Temperaturregulation. Urban und Schwarzenberg, Munich
46 Isbruch FM, Koch T, Greve H, Dittrich H, Heuer H (1988) Die zentralvenöse Bluttemperatur als Sensor für ein frequenzadaptives Schrittmachersystem. Biomed Tech (Berlin) 33:295–299
47 Koch T, Isbruch FM, Frenking B, Greve H, Gülker H, Heuer H (1988) Longterm results with the temperature controlled pacemaker Thermos 01. PACE 11 (Cardiostim 88):807
48 Laczkovics A, Simbrunner G, Losert U (1982) Temperaturmessungen zur Steuerung der Herzfrequenz in der Schrittmacherchirurgie. Kongressbericht Osterr Ges Chir 23:119
49 Fearnot NE, Evans ML (1988) Heart rate correlation, response time and effect of previous exercise using an advanced pacing rate algorithm for temperature-based rate modulation. PACE 11:1846–1852
50 Griffin JC, Jutzy KR, Claude JP, Knutti JW (1983) Central body temperature as a guide to optimal heart rate. PACE 6:498–501
51 Laczkovics A, Laufer G, Oehner T, Schlich W (1987) First clinical results with a temperature guided rate responsive pacemaker. PACE 10:1216
52 Naumann d'Alnoncourt C, Schnabel F, Baumann B, Helwing HP (1987) Temperaturgesteuerter Herzschrittmacher THERMOS 01 nach His-Bündel Ablation. Herzschrittmacher 7:168–174
53 Schaldach M (1989) Herzschrittmacher mit temperaturgesteuerter Frequenzanpassung. Herzschrittmacher 9:5–14
54 Schaldach M (1988) Compensation of chronotropic incompetence with temperature-controlled rate adaptive pacing. Biomed Tech (Berlin) 33:286–294
55 Ulmer HV (1987) Arbeitsphysiology. In: Schmidt RF, Thews G (eds) Physiologie des Menschen, 23rd edn. Springer, Berlin Heidelberg New York, pp 683–704
56 Wassermann K (1966) Interactions of physiological mechanisms during exercise. J Appl Physiol 22:71–85
57 Rickards AF, Norman J (1981) Relation between QT interval and heart rate. New design of physiologically adaptive cardiac pacemaker. Br Heart J 45:56
58 Kékes E, Mihóczy L (1989) Systolic and diastolic time intervals. In: Ghista DN, Mihóczy L (eds) Noninvasive cardiac assessment technology. Karger, Basel, pp 47–55
59 Rentsch W (1980) Technical aspects for acquisition of systolic time intervals especially for determination of the preejection index. In: List WF, Gravenstein IS, Spodick DH (eds) Systolic time intervals. Springer Berlin Heidelberg New York, pp 133–141
60 Ross J, Sobel BE (1972) Regulation of cardiac contraction. Ann Rev Physiol 34:47–90
61 Spodick DH, Doi YL, Bishop RL, Hashimoto T (1984) Systolic time intervals reconsidered – reevaluation of the preejection period absence of relation to heart rate. Am J Cardiol 53:1667–1670
62 Weissler AM (1974) Noninvasive cardiology. Grune & Stratton, New York
63 Smith JJ, Muzi M, Barney JA, Ceschi J, Hayes J, Ebert TJ (1989) Impedance-derived cardiac indices in supine and upright exercise. Ann Biomed Eng 17:507–515
64 Chirife R (1988) Physiological principles of a new method for rate responsive pacing using the preejection interval. Pace 11:1545–1554
65 Niederlag W, Rentsch W, Wunderlich E, Schmidt PKH (1989) Ist die Anspannungszeit ein brauchbarer Parameter für die frequenzadaptierte Herzstimulation? Biomed Tech (Berlin) 34 (Suppl):62–65
66 Rentsch W, Niederlag W, Foelske H, Wunderlich E, Schmidt PKH (1987) Zur physiologi-

schen Frequenzanpassung von Herzschrittmachern mittels systolischer Zeitintervalle. Z Gesamte Inn Med 42:386–389
67 Salo RW, Pederson BD, Olive AL, Lincoln WC, Wallner TG (1984) Continuous ventricular volume assessment for diagnosis and pacemaker control. PACE 7:1267–1272
68 Schaldach M (1989) Systolic time intervals as a control of rate adaptive pacing. Proc IEEE Eng Med Biol 11:1407–1410
69 Kubicek WG (1989) On the source of peak first time derivative (dZ/dt) during impedance cardiography. Ann Biomed Eng 17:459–462
70 Kubicek WG, Patterson RP, Witsoe DA (1970) Impedance cardiography as a noninvasive method of monitoring cardiac function and other parameters of the cardiovascular system. Ann NY Acad Sci 170:724–732
71 Geddes LA, Hoff HE, Mellow A, Palmer C (1966) Continuous measurement of ventricular stroke volume by electrical impedance. Cardiac Res Center Bull 4:118–130
72 Baan J, van der Velde ET, Stenndijk P, Koops J (1989) Calibration and application of the conductance catheter for ventricular volume measurement. In: Valentinuzzi ME (ed) Intracardiac conductance volumetry. Gordon and Breach, New York, pp 357–365 (Automedica, vol II)
73 Herrera MC, Clavin OE, Spinelli JC, Valentinuzzi ME, Cabrera Fischer EI, Pichel RH (1986) Multichannel tetrapolar admittance meter (MY) for intracardiac volume measurments in animals. Med Prog Technol 11:43–49
74 McKay RG, Spears JR, Aroesty JM, Baim DS, Royal HD, Heller GV, Lincoln W, Salo RW, Braunwald E, Grossmann W (1984) Instantaneous measurement of left and right ventricular volume and pressure-volume relationships with an impedance catheter. Circulation 69:703–710
75 Woodard JC, Bertram CD, Gow BS (1987) Right ventricular volumetry by catheter measurement of conductance. PACE 10:862–870
76 Schaldach M, Rentsch W, Rentsch HW (1990) Advances in intracardiac impedance plethysmography. Proc IEEE Eng Med Biol 12/2:711–713
77 Schaldach M (1989) PEP-gesteuerter Herzschrittmacher. Biomed Tech (Berlin) 34:177–184
78 Boheim G, Schaldach M (1988) Frequenzadaption eines künstlichen Herzschrittmachers über einen Volumenregelkreis. Biomed Tech (Berlin) 33:100–105
79 Boheim G (1988) Intrakardiale Impedanzmessung zur frequenzadaptiven Stimulation des Herzens. Dissertation, Zentralinstitut für Biomedizinische Technik, Erlangen.

# Safety Standards for Cardiac Pacemakers

N. LEITGEB

## Introduction

Although reliability and safety testing of cardiac pacemakers in Austria is not obligatory, it is stated by law that every electrical device on the market has to fulfill all relevant safety regulations and standards. Not to meet those requirements, therefore, constitutes a legal violation which may force the responsible ministry to find the company and prohibit the sale of the device in Austria. Austrian safety standards for electromedical equipment are harmonized with CENELEC standards. General requirements include ÖVE-MG/IEC 601–1 [9], which is the equivalent of the European HD 395.1S2 (1988) and IEC 601–1 (1977 + 1984) [3, 6]. For implantable cardiac pacemakers EN 50061 (1988) and ISO 5841–1 (1989) contain supplementary requirements [4, 5]. The intention of these standards is to protect patients from hazards. Yet at the same time, they are not so cumbersome as to restrict the development of new devices. Standards in effect at this time specifiy: (1) packaging, labeling, and documentation as to intended use/restriction on the device; (2) measures taken to protect against electrical hazards; (3) measures taken to protect against malfunction.

## Tolerance Specifications

Austrian and other applicable standards define certain parameters and nominal values to be met by all cardiac pacemakers. Tolerance limits which must be met are specified by the manufacturers in literature supplied with each unit. Tolerances so specified include:

1. Stimulus duration (ms), measured between the 30% points of the ascending and descending slopes of the pacing stimulus
2. Stimulus amplitude (V or mA), i.e., the arithmetic mean value for pacing stimulus amplitude averaged over the stimulus duration time
3. Basic pulse interval (ms), i.e., the time between two consecutive pacing stimuli in the absence of sensed cardiac events or electromechanical interference
4. Basc rate (paced pulses/min-ppm), i.e., the mean pulse rate in the absence of sensed cardiac events or during electromagnetic interference, determined as the inverse of the mean value of 20 basic pulse intervals (60 000/mean value)
5. Sensitivity (mV), i.e., the minimum peak amplitude of a specified test impulse that

can be sensed by the pacemaker and definded for both positive (e positive) and negative (e negative) impulses

6. Input impedance (ohms), defined as the impedance measured with a specified test impulse between the active and neutral poles of the pacemaker
7. Escape interval (ms), which is the time between a simulated sensed beat and the succeeding, nontriggered pacing stimulus
8. Refractory period (ms), which is the time after stimulation during which simulated beats do not lead to pacemaker responses. According to the type of pacemaker, one may differentiate a sensing refractory period, a stimulation refractory period (inhibited pacemakers only), or both.

A functional disturbance (malfunction) is defined as deviation of any of the aforementioned parameters from the manufacturer's specified tolerance range. Malfunction could be due to, for example, external effects such as electromagnetic interference.

## Technical Requirements for Pacemakers

### *Protection During Transport and Storage*

Pacemakers must be supplied in a sterilized package in such a manner that they can withstand all mechanical and thermal stresses occasioned by normal handling during transport and storage without loss of sterility or reliability of function. For example, pacemakers must withstand defined mechanical shocks and vibration without loss of compliance with the requirements (EN 50061) [4]. Pacemakers must remain functional after exposure to temperatures between 0°C and 50°C (EN 50061).

### *Protection to the Patient*

Pacemakers must be constructed in such a manner that their presence within the body does not lead to harmful biological consequences. Thus, standards are set for:

1. Biocompatibility: Pacemaker parts in direct contact with body tissues or fluids must be of biocompatible material, i.e., material that does not produce adverse tissue reactions or cell mutations.
2. Electrical safety: Except for their intended function, pacemakers must be essentially electrically neutral if implanted. Since no ideal insulating materials are available, leakage currents to the surrounding tissue are unavoidable. To prevent excessive electrolytic effects, D.C. leakage currents must not exceed 100 nA.
3. Stimulation rate safety: "Run-away" protection from excessive stimulation rates must be ensured by limiting the maximum possible stimulation rate.
4. Mechanical safety: Pacemakers must be constructed to withstand mechanical vibration occasioned by walking, jogging, cycling, driving, etc.
5. End of service indicator: There must be some means by which noninvasive detection of impending battery (power source) depletion is possible, as well as some indication of the actual battery status.

6. Model identification: A radiopaque code must be provided, enabling the physician to identify the manufacturer and model of a particular pacemaker following implantation.

*Protection Against Pacemaker Malfunction*

Every pacemaker with its sensing electrode forms a system which, like an antenna, is able to receive signals from different sources. Electrodes, therefore, not only sense intrinsic cardiac activity but also electromagnetic and other interference which could affect pacemaker function or even damage the pacemaker system. The sensitivity to interference differs between different types of pacemaker systems and electrode configurations. Bipolar electrodes are the least susceptible to interference, and unipolar electrodes the most susceptible. The greater the distance between a unipolar electrode and the pacer pulse generator ("can") itself, the greater the likelihood of poor interference performance. Therefore, unipolar electrodes should be as close as possible to the pacer can. To wind or stack electrode leads around the pacer can does not reduce the antenna effect.

Depending on the antenna potential for a particular pacemaker lead system and the frequency of the interfering signal, any or all the following effects may occur:

1. Direct thermal myocardial damage with current densities exceeding some $mA/cm^2$ [dependent on tissue properties, temporal exposure characteristic, and "crest factor" (the peak to average ratio of a signal)] which may occur at the small electrode tip due to induction by strong high frequency energy sources.".
2. Fibrillation with current densities exceeding 100 $\mu A/cm^2$.
3. Irreversible damage to the pulse generator electronics or program changes due to induced voltages.
4. Reversible, functional myocardial changes due to induced voltages. These will depend on the amplitude of the interference signal. Interference signals with amplitudes greater than those of myocardial signals may cause the pacemaker to revert to asynchronous operation (interference mode) at some specified rate. With the cessation of interference, the pacemaker returns to its previously programmed mode of operation without further adjustment. Alternatively, interference signals may be interpreted as myocardial signals causing inappropriate triggering/inhibition of pulse generator output.
5. Interference signals with amplitudes lower than those of the expected myocardial potentials should not affect pacemaker function.

The potential for harm to the patient is greatest in the following situations. First, with asynchronous pacing in the interference mode, pacing occurs without regard to the existing spontaneous activity of the heart. If, as a consequence, there is interference with the heart's native rhythm, parasystole may occur. Parasystole may lead to a reduction in cardiac output, which can be the cause for dizziness or syncope. Nevertheless, due to relatively low pacing energies the risk of fibrillation is generally low, with the qualification that with preexisting pathophysiology or acute reduced acid-base or electrolyte imbalance fibrillation thresholds may be reduced. Second, if the interference signal is misinterpreted as native heart activity interference may cause pacemaker inhibition and asystole. This may be the cause of dizziness or syncope only if it coincides with a sufficiently long duration of native heart inactivity. On the other hand, interference signals may lead to inappropriate triggering of pacemaker output, thereby increasing the paced rate. With modern pacemakers, however, pacemaker output is limited by a preset or programmed upper rate limit (typically 150 ppm). Although the risk of such pacemaker interference has been estimated differently [2, 7, 10], there is no doubting the potential importance of interference events in daily life. For example, in one series of patients monitored by 24-hour Holter ECG, 83% of patients were observed to have some sort of pacemaker malfunction due to interference. The frequency of such occurrences was between 1 and 110 events per day [2].

The following types of electromagnetic interference can be identified:

1. Endogenous events (e.g., myopotentials)
2. Medical and diagnostic therapy, including defibrillation, electrotherapy, diathermy, electrocautery, radiation therapy, extracorporeal shock wave lithotripsy, diagnostic x-rays, nuclear magnetic resonance imaging
3. Ambient electromagnetic sources, including leakage currents from electrical devices, sensor switches, extra low frequency electric and magnetic fields from high tension lines and electrical devices, and radio frequency emissions from automatic door opening or alarm systems and radio or television stations.

Due to ongoing controversies, it has not yet been possible to reach international agreement on the technical requirements for electromagnetic compatibility of pacemaker systems. The initial aim, to be able to provide reasonable assurance that a pacemaker patient will be at no greater risk from ambient electromagnetic fields than a person without a pacemaker, has not been achieved in draft proposals presented up to now. Draft proposonal to present define two electromagnetic signal interference levels. Below the first, the pacemaker system will remain unaffected and function in its set mode. In between the two levels, the system will operate as intended or change to an asynchronous interference mode, with return to initial set mode function (without additional adjustment) after the termination of electromagnetic interference. Finally, electromagnetic interference with amplitudes above the second level may cause irreversible and/or undefined functional changes to the pacemaker system.

Ambient electric and magnetic fields of sufficient strength can cause adverse effects in patients with pacemakers (Fig. 1). Therefore the International Radiation Protection Agency, in cooperation with the World Health Organization, has developed guidelines on limits of exposure to 50- to 60-Hz electric and magnetic fields for the general public. Besides this, a few countries have already established or are about to establish national limits for exposure. Figure 1 shows that the established limits will provide some margin of safety against adverse biological effects. However, existing or recommended exposure limits for patients with pacemakers will not necessarily protect the patient from possible adverse effects on pacemaker function. There may be an even greater danger of adverse effects on pacemaker operation in the workplace, where exposure limits may be raised fivefold over those for nonworking environments.

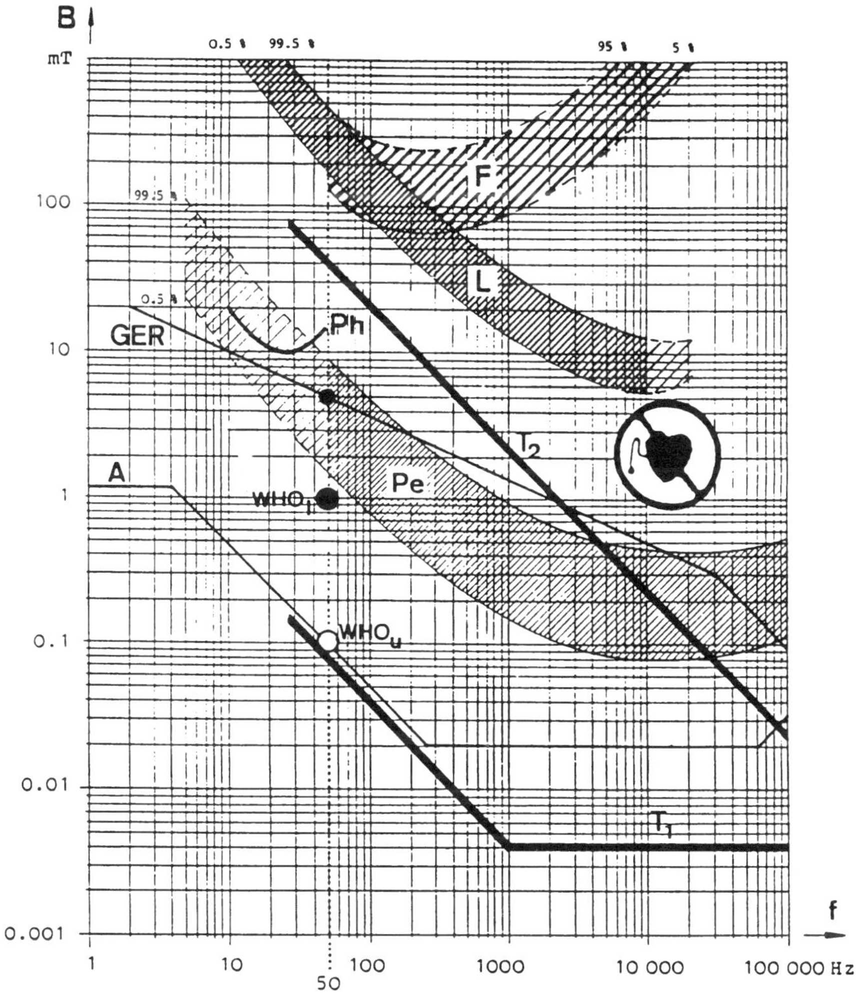


**Fig. 1.** Interaction of extremely low frequency magnetic field in people with implanted pacemakers. *mT*, millitesla; *F*, fibrillation; *L*, let-go-threshold (total excitation of skeletal muscle); *Ph*, magnetophosphenes (excitation of the retina); *Pe*, perception threshold (cellular stimulation); *GER*, exposure limit in Germany (unlimited duration); *A*, recommended exposure limit in Austria (unlimited duration); $WHO_l$, recommended exposure limit, Word Health Organization (duration limited to a few hours per day); $WHO_u$, recommended exposure limit, World Health Organization (unlimited duration); $T_1$, limit for uninfluenced action of pacemakers; $T_2$, limit for irreversible and/or undefined effects on pacemaker operation

## Summary

Austrian safety standards for cardiac pacemakers are harmonized with the CENELEC and IEC standards. Standards specify measures for product identification to prevent electrical and biocompatibily hazards and malfunction. Details on technical requirements for pacemakers are given. Due to ongoing controversies, international agreement on the technical requirements for electromagnetic compatibility of pacemaker systems has not yet been reached. Implanting physicians as well as the patient should be aware of the potential importance of interference events in daily life. Therefore pacemaker systems with minimum interference sensitivity are to be preferred and the pacer pulse generator should be implanted as close as possible to the electrodes, with electrode leads as short as possible. Patients should be informed as to the potential interference sources, the characteristic interference behaviour of their pacemaker system, and the symptoms they might experience with pacemaker interference.

## References

1 Bethge KP, Brandes A, Gonska BD (1989) Diagnostic sensitivity of Holter monitoring in pacemaker patients. J Ambul Monitoring 2:79–89
2 Bossert T, Dahme M (1988) Hazards from electromagnetic fields: influence on cardiac pacemakers. IERE Publ 81:13–18
3 Cenelec HD 395.1S2 (1988) Medical electrical equipment. Part 1: General requirements
4 EN 50061 (July 1988) Safety of implantable pacemakers. European standard
5 EN 50061 prA1 (1991) Safety of implantable pacemakers. Draft proposal on protection against electrical magnetic interference. Draft European standard
6 IEC 601–1 (1988) Medical electrical equipment, 2nd edn. Part 1: General requirements for safety
7 Irnich W (1988) Herzschrittmacher und nichtionisierende Strahlung. Proceedings Nichtionisierende Strahlung, Cologne, pp 162–169
8 Leitgeb N (1990) Strahlen, Wellen, Felder. Ursachen und Auswirkung auf Umwelt und Gesundheit. Thieme Stuttgart
9 ÖVE-MG/IEC 601 (1986) Sicherheit elektromedizinischer Geräte. Part 1: Allgemeine Bestimmungen
10 Silny J (1988) Störbeeinflussung von Herzschrittmachern durch magnetische Wechselfelder. Proceedings Nichtionisierende Strahlung, Cologne, pp 170–172
11 WHO/IRPA/INIRC (1988) Interim guidelines on limits of exposure to 50/60 Hz electric and magnetic fields. Health Physics 58:113–122

# Prevention of Crosstalk in Dual Chamber Pacemakers

H. BROUWER AND J.W.J. VAN HOVE

## Definitions

Atrioventricular crosstalk in dual chamber pacemakers is when the atrial stimulus is sensed by the ventricular sensing amplifier, leading to inhibition of ventricular output [1]. With atrioventricular (AV) crosstalk, for example, a 5 V stimulus from the atrial channel might be sensed as a small (0.3 V) artefact by the QRS detector (Fig. 1).

A ventricular sensing amplifier consists of an input filter and amplification circuit (Fig. 2). With an output amplitude of 5 V at the atrial channel, there is the possibility

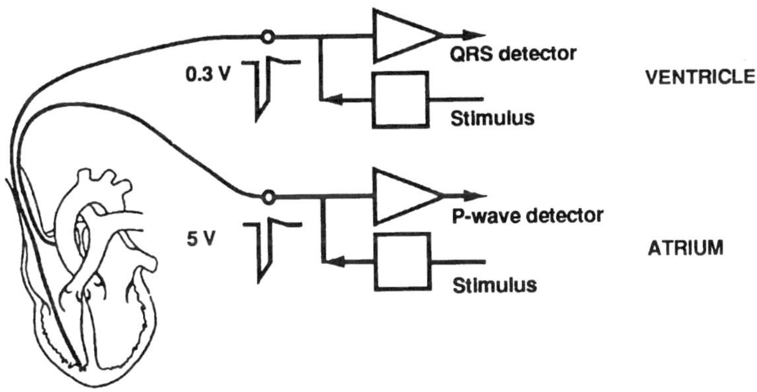


**Fig. 1.** Atrioventricular crosstalk. A 5 V atrial stimulus is sensed as a 0.3 V artefact by the QRS detector (sensing channel), leading to inhibition of ventricular output.

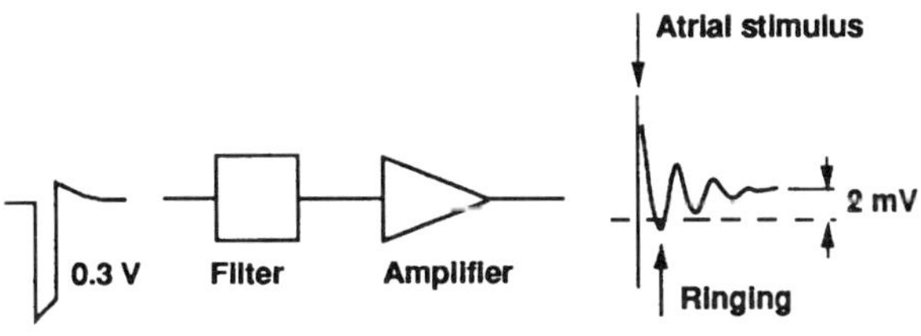


**Fig. 2.** Ventricular sensing amplifier. Ringing (see text) following the sensed atrial pacing stimulus leads to inhibition of ventricular output; that is, ringing is interpreted as a QRS complex.

of measuring approximately 0.3 V at the ventricular sensing amplifier. Due to "ringing" at the ventricular amplifier which occurs when a large amplitude signal is applied to a very sensitive sensing amplifier, the atrial stimulus artefact might be detected as a normal QRS.

## Clinical Example

A clinical illustration of crosstalk for an AV universal (DDD) pacemaker is provided in Fig. 3. In this ECG recording from a patient with complete (third degree) AV block and an implanted DDD pacemaker, with crosstalk there is stimulation of the atrium

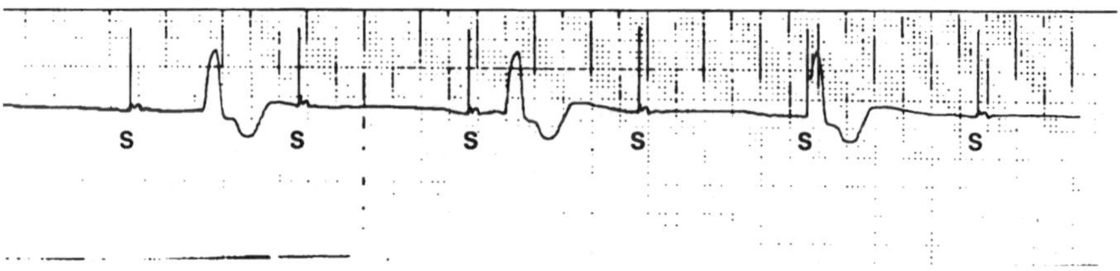


**Fig. 3.** ECG strip illustrating AV crosstalk. Atrial pacing stimuli (**S**) are sensed by ventricular sensing amplifier, leading to inhibition of ventricular output. Pacing stimuli bear no relation to QRS and the fifth such stimulus falls within the QRS complex

but no ventricular stimulus after the programmed AV delay of 160 ms (Fig. 3). Additionally, there is no sensing of a spontaneous QRS because the ventricular sensing amplifier is refractory after having sensed crosstalk artefact produced by the atrial stimulus.

## Technical Solutions

Several factors will influence the likelihood of crosstalk with dual-chamber pacemakers. The use of a bipolar as opposed to a unipolar ventricular electrode can reduce the incidence of crosstalk. For example, if with a unipolar electrode the crosstalk artefact is approximately 0.3 V, sensing with a bipolar electrode will diminish this artefact to a level of 50 mV. But even a 50 mV artefact entering a ventricular sensing amplifier programmed to a 2 mV sensitivity level will be detected and interpreted as a normal QRS. While the atrial output can be programmed to a lower output setting, this is less effective than reprogramming the ventricular sensitivity to a higher value. Such reprogramming, however, will not always prevent crosstalk.

Further, the location of the ventricular electrode will also affect the likelihood of crosstalk. An electrode located at the apex of the right ventricle, as opposed to near the pulmonary outflow track, will be less apt to sense an atrial pacing stimulus or polarization artefact.

These technical solutions for prevention of crosstalk in DDD pacemakers will not eliminate the problem in all patients. This is compounded by the fact that 80% of European electrode implants are of unipolar configuration.[1] Therefore, only correct programming of atrial output and ventricular sensitivity can help to improve prevention of crosstalk.

## Programming Solution

Programming solutions such as providing a "blanking period" (ventricular sensing amplifier refractory to any signals for a specified time after the atrial stimulus) must be adapted to meet individual patient requirements. This can be a difficult and time-consuming procedure.

In addition to the blanking technique, safety or window pacing offers an alternative, and possibly better, means of protection against crosstalk. With safety pacing, ventricular pacing is committed, i.e., any post-blanking period sensing by the ventricular sensing amplifier will not inhibit ventricular output. Therefore, with safety pacing, the ventricular channel will always stimulate the ventricle after an atrial stimulus, with the possibility of stimulation during a spontaneous ventricular beat to produce a fusion or pseudofusion QRS complex.

## Retriggerable Window

Automatic adjustment of the blanking period (without additional programming) and full reliability of sensing would provide the optimum solution for prevention of crosstalk. One such solution is termed the "retrigerabble window" (Fig. 4). With the retriggerable window, the atrial stimulus initiates a blanking interval which is a little longer than the ringing interval of the ventricular amplifier. During the retriggerable window, sensing of ventricular signals will not cause inhibition of the ventricular

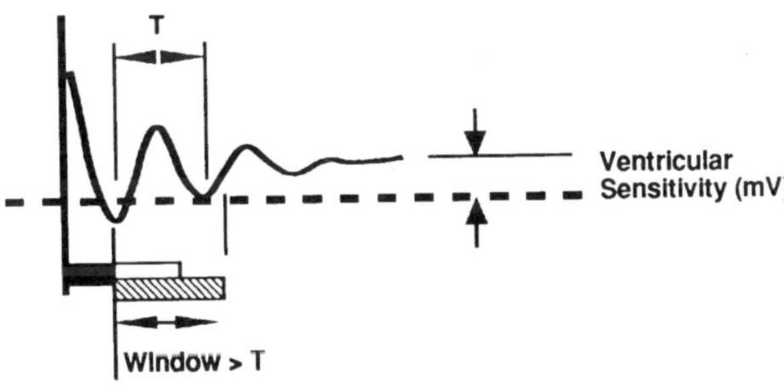


**Fig. 4.** Retriggerable window. *T* denotes one periodic ringing interval. See text for further discussion

[1]Editors note (J.L.A.): In the United States, approximately 60% (the trend is upward) of current Medtronic electrode sales of DDD pacemakers are for the bipolar configuration (Edwin G. Duffin, PhD, Medtronic, personal communication).

stimulus but will restart (retrigger) the window. The ringing period of any amplifier is fully determined by the filter characteristics of the amplifier. These are known because the amplifier is built with fixed components. During this ringing interval, artefact will retrigger the sensing window. If there is no detection of another artefact, inhibition of ventricular output is possible as soon as the window ends. If an artefact has occurred during this window, the blanking period of the ventricular sensing amplifier will be extended automatically.

Thus, the objective of preventing crosstalk in DDD pacemakers is achieved by providing a retriggerable window. Provision of the retriggerable window results in short blanking periods when no or little crosstalk is present. However, if conditions are favourable for crosstalk, the blanking period or retriggerable window will automatically be longer. To date 4000 Vitatron DDD pacemakers with the "retriggerable window" crosstalk prevention feature built in have been implanted. No cases of crosstalk disturbance have been reported for these patients. (Technical date on file with "Vitatron Medical B.V.").

## Summary

Atrioventricular crosstalk is ventricular sensing of atrial stimulation artefact or depolarization leading to inhibition of a ventricular output. The use of bipolar lead configurations will reduce but not entirely limit crosstalk in dual chamber pacemakers, as can location of ventricular leads at the right ventricular apex. Programming solutions to reduce crosstalk include provision of a blanking period and/or safety pacing. Finally, optimum solution for prevention of crosstalk may be the retriggerable window, incorporated in recent models of Vitatron DDD pacemakers.

## References

1 Barold S, Ong L, Falkoff M, Heinle R (1985) Crosstalk or self-inhibition in dual-chambered pacemakers . In: Barold S (ed) Modern cardiac pacing. Futura, New York, pp 615–623

# Modern Pacemakers

R. SUTTON

## Introduction

Cardiac pacing can bring dramatic clinical benefit to patients with bradycardia. It represents the first sucessful application of electronic technology to medical therapy. Implanted pacing systems have been in use for over 30 years [1]. Recent times have seen increasing sophistication in an attempt to produce both an appropriate heart rate for every clinical occasion and to maintain the normal atrioventricular (AV) sequence. By so doing, modern pacemakers mimic normal sinus rhythm.

## Pacemakers

A basic or single chamber pacemaker has one pacing lead connecting it to one cardiac chamber, usually the right ventricle. It has one stimulation rate, but since the late 1960s has incorporated an additional detection circuit for spontaneous heart activity: this is known as demand function. The pacing lead, when it detects a spontaneous beat, resets the timing clock within the generator so that the ventricular output stimulus is withheld. This permits periods of normal cardiac rhythm to inhibit the output of the pacemaker, leaving it on standby to intervene only if normal rhythm fails. Such a pacemaker is known as ventricular demand or inhibited VVI [2]; that is, the system paces the ventricles (V), detects spontaneous activity in the ventricles (V) and responds to detected activity by inhibition (I) of stimulus output. The advent of the silicon chip and other technologies, such as small, high capacity lithium batteries and external programming by radio frequency communication links, has allowed much more flexibility to be built into single chamber pacemakers. Concurrent with the increase in complexity, there has been an increase in reliability. Pacemaker programmability enables the physician to adjust rate, output (voltage/current and pulse duration), sensitivity and refractory periods, and to apply rate hysteresis. Rate hysteresis is a valuable feature which maximizes the opportunity for spontaneous cardiac rhythm to inhibit pacemaker output. This is achieved by setting the generator to be inhibited by spontaneous rates which are less than its automatic pacing rate. For example, 50 bpm may be set as the hysteresis rate which triggers pulse generator output. When spontaneous activity falls below 50 bpm, the pulse generator stimulates the heart at 70 bpm (automatic rate). Thus, the pacing system will not intervene during sleep, when many patients have a slow but haemodynamically adequate rhythm.

## Rate Responsive Pacemakers

During the past decade, many models of pacemakers have incorporated the ability to vary the rate of stimulation in accordance with patient's activity — sitting, walking, sleeping, etc. Initially this was achieved by use of an additional right atrial lead connected for detection of P waves [3]. Upon detection the generator allows an AV delay (equivalent to a PR interval) and then paces the right ventricle. In many pacemaker recipients with AV block atrial activity is normal and responds normally to autonomic nervous system regulation. Atrial sensing with triggering of ventricular output (VAT) after some preset or programmed AV interval, therefore, provides an imitation of the normal sinus mechanism for the patient who has AV block. During exercise, the atrial rate is faster and the paced ventricular rate rises with it. During sleep, the atrial rate is naturally slow; hence the ventricular stimulation rate is slower. Another type of pacemaker (VDD) paces only the ventricle (V) but senses both the atria and the ventricles (D for dual). Since it has two sensing responses — that is, atrial sensing triggers ventricular output except that a sensed ventricular event before the end of a preset/programmed AV interval inhibits ventricular output — the letter D in the third position indicates dual sensing response. Soon thereafter, such units were also given the ability to pace in the atria if the atrial rate fell below the basic pacemaker rate, thereby providing dual chamber stimulation capacity (D). Such pacers are termed AV universal or DDD.

In the early 1980s an alternative concept of rate variability or rate modulation developed. Two factors led to this development. First, a desire to keep the pacing system simple and to stimulate only one pair of chambers with only one lead. Second, to provide rate variability even in the event of abnormal atrial function (little or no increase in atrial rate with exertion — termed chronotropic incompetence) or of atrial fibrillation. The original approach was to use the stimulating electrode for sensing the duration of the stimulus-T interval [4]. This was shown to be influenced by circulating catecholamines, shortening with increased concentrations. Two other sensors were devised in the early 1980s to detect changes in respiratory rate with exercise. The first measured changes in chest wall impedance by passing a small current between an additional subcutaneous lead and the pulse generator. The second sensed vibration by means of a piezoelectric crystal inside the pulse generator. The latter system, known as activity sensing, proved most simple and efficacious to use in combination with rate responsive ventricular pacemakers (VVIR). More recently, temperature sensing using a thermistor on the pacing lead, right ventricular pressure sensing using a piezoelectric crystal on the pacing lead, and respiratory minute volume sensing by measurement of chest wall impedance and fibreoptic assessment of venous oxygen saturation have all been tested [5]. At present, the most widely used sensor is activity sensing, which type of sensor has how been combined with DDD pacemakers to provide dual chamber rate responsive pacing (DDDR). This offers the benefit of AV sequential pacing to patients with AV block, but also with an attenuated sinus node response to exercise. Rate responsive DDD pacemakers [6] are still in an early stage of evaluation.

## Benefits of Rate Responsive Pacemakers

Cardiologists began their assessment of technological advances for VDD pacemakers with haemodynamic studies. They soon became more interested in exercise testing, especially when the second generation of VDD pacemakers could also be programmed to the VVI mode. This offered the possibility of within-patient comparisons of pacing modes. Studies in the early 1980s showed an approximate 25% gain in cardiac output and exercise capacity with VDD compared to VVI pacing [7, 8]. The studies that followed were even more interesting because they focused on the quality of life benefits of physiological (rate-adaptive) stimulation versus single rate ventricular pacing [9]. All these studies were conducted in patients with AV block, but with normal sinus node function. Rate responsive VVI pacemakers (VVIR) could also be programmed back to the VVI mode so that comparisons could be made between the two modes. Such comparisons have been made with many different types of sensor systems. Results have shown some benefit in terms of maximum exercise capacity [10]. They have also shown increases in peak oxygen consumption and anaerobic threshold with the rate responsive mode [11]. Results of assessment of the benefit in terms of quality of life have been less clear cut than those of comparisons between the VDD and VVI pacing modes [12]. With the advent of DDDR pacemakers, comparisons of DDDR and DDD, DDD and VVIR, and other modes are now in progress. It is of great importance that rate responsive pacing technology undergoes vigorous clinical scrutiny before more widespread adoption.

With autonomic nervous system disorders affecting heart rate control (carotid sinus and vasovagal syndromes), there is little or no disease of conduction tissue and the heart usually responds to exercise in a normal way [13, 14]. However, during syncopal attacks with these conditions, there is always some element of peripheral vasodilatation (vasodepression). Thus, not only is there cardioinhibition but also rapidly falling venous return. At such times dual chamber stimulation is required to maximize cardiac output. Atrial stimulation is untenable because of vagally mediated conduction slowing at the atrioventricular node. Ventricular stimulation alone may be haemodynamically ineffective. Further, if retrograde AV conduction occurs, it may actually be counterproductive, especially if atrial systole coincides with ventricular systole. When this happens, the atria contract against closed AV valves and blood is regurgitated into the pulmonary and systemic veins, leading to reduced ventricular preload in the subsequent diastole.

Retrograde AV conduction is the usual mechanism for the pacemaker syndrome [15], one of the chief side-effects of ventricular pacing. It occurs in approximately 20% of patients with VVI pacing; about half of these are overtly symptomatic with palpitations, dyspnoea, findings of heart failure, and occasionally renewed dizziness and syncope, while the remainder have more subtle symptoms and findings. All patients may substantially benefit by conversion of their pacing systems to atrial or dual chamber pacing, as appropriate for the patient's electrophysiology (i.e. bradycardia due to AV conduction block or sinus node dysfunction).

Atrial natriuretic peptide (ANP) is elevated in venous blood with increased atrial stretch [16]. With chronic DDD pacing, the concentrations of ANP are not significantly different from normals of similar age [17]. However, the same patients programmed to VVI will increase their ANP concentrations to over twice normal values, and those with the pacemaker syndrome can have greater than three times normal values [18]. Patients with VVIR pacemakers will have lower levels of ANP during exercise compared to patients with VVI pacers [19]. These data lend further support to the more physiological nature of rate adaptive pacing.

## Conditions for Which Pacing is Indicated

### *Atrioventricular Block*

Pacing is most effective in conditions which are associated with presyncopal dizziness or syncope. The best known of these is AV block. When this presents as complete AV block with syncope, the decision to implant a permanent pacing system is relatively clear cut. However, there are patients who present with fatigue or heart failure, or in whom bradycardia is documented, and are shown to have complete AV block. These patients might also require pacing since they could at any time experience bradycardiac arrest, with the potential for mortality or morbidity from injuries sustained consequent to syncopal attacks. There are also patients who have intermittent AV block or a lesser degree of AV block who can present with normal sinus rhythm. Usually there is some evidence of AV conduction system disease, which may be apparent as bundle branch block possibly combined with an increase in the PR interval. Such patients with AV conduction system disease require further investigation for sinus node competence. An exercise test and 24-hour electrocardiography (ECG) may be sufficient. Results of this testing will influence the pacing mode choice. With normal sinus node function, the VDD or DDD modes are optimal. If there is abnormal sinus node function, the DDD mode is advised. In some patients, the sino-atrial node may fail to increase its rate above 100 bpm during maximal exercise testing. For these patients, a new mode of sensor-driven rate responsive dual chamber pacing (DDDR) should be considered, unless there is chronic atrial fibrillation associated with AV block. Atrial fibrillation prevents any form of pacing or sensing in the atria. With atrial fibrillation, an exercise test will reveal the ability of the ventricles to increase their rate. If such ability is suboptimal or absent, the VVIR mode of pacing is ideal; if it is present, the VVI mode should be adequate.

With intermittent AV block, even more detailed investigation may be required, including a cardiac electrophysiologic study with His bundle recording to determine the exact site of AV conduction defects. Of particular interest is the duration of the His to ventricular activation time. The normal value is 35–55 ms. Values above 100 ms are widely accepted as being of pathological significance. With a history strongly suggestive of cardiac syncope but negative electrophysiological findings, some authorities employ stress pacing [20] or intravenous antiarrhythmic drugs such as ajmaline [21] or flecainide [22]. If, with these interventions, the His-ventricular interval extends to 100 ms or more, it is inferred that there is a high possibility of subsequent AV block and that the patient's presenting symptoms were also due to AV block.

Atrioventricular block carries a mortality of approximately 50% in 5 years [23]. This can be reduced to 5%–15% with institution of pacing [24]. It is possible that dual chamber pacing (VDD or DDD) will ultimately be shown to provide the lowest mortality [25]. The aetiology of acquired AV block in Western countries is most frequently (40%) an idiopathic patchy fibrosis involving the conduction tissue [26]. Other important causes are coronary artery disease (15%), cardiomyopathy (15%) and aortic valve disease with calcification (5%). AV block can also complicate cardiac surgery, especially with closure of ventricular septal defects or replacement of the aortic valve. The sex distribution is even and the average age of presentation of AV block is 70 years [27].

Congenital AV block is most commonly due to conduction block at the level of the AV node [28]. It is therefore most often associated with an AV junctional pacemaker, a narrow complex QRS ($\leq 0.12$ s) and the ability to increase ventricular rate with exertion. These patients usually present at a young age. Some will benefit from pacing even at a young age, especially if there is an inadequate ventricular rate increase with exercise or 24-hour ECG shows complex ventricular extrasystoles for which antiarrhythmic therapy is required. All antiarrhythmic drugs should be considered to have the potential to depress conduction below the AV node and produce inadequate ventricular escape rhythms.

*Sick Sinus Syndrome*

Sick sinus syndrome is of unknown aetiology in the majority of patients. Histologically, it is associated with patchy fibrosis throughout the atria [29]. The sex distribution is even and the average age at presentation is 70 years. Sick sinus syndrome is a common condition in the elderly, but only a small proportion of the patients present with dizziness, syncope or heart failure that can be attributed to bradycardia [30]. At present these are the only patients who should be considered for permanent pacing [31]. In my opinion sick sinus syndrome is often quite difficult to diagnose because a complex array of findings is required. There may be obvious sino-atrial block or sinus arrest on the resting ECG, but more often 24-hour ECGs are required. The lack of a tachycardiac response to exercise or intravenous atropine provides further confirmation. Electrophysiological tests of sinus node function are frequently presented as additional evidence. The most commonly used of these tests is sinus node recovery time. With this test, the sinus node is overdriven by rapid atrial pacing. Then the spontaneous sinus interval is subtracted from the time interval to the first spontaneous, sinus-origin beat following cessation of pacing [32]. Direct recordings of the sinus node activity itself have also been made but are not routinely done. Occasionally the intrinsic heart rate is determined in the presence of pharmacologic autonomic blockade with propranolol and atropine [33]. It is possible that intravenous antiarrhythmic drugs may also be used as a stress test of sinus node function, similar to testing of AV conduction. Flecainide is probably the most valuable drug in this context [22]. With cessation of sinus automaticity or sino-atrial exit block, atrial tachyarrhythmias can occur (bradycardia-tachycardia syndrome). This is not surprising since in most cases of sinus node disease the atria are also diseased, providing the substrate for ectopic or re-entrant atrial tachyarrhythmias. Thus, not only are bradycardias features of sick sinus syndrome but so too are atrial tachyarrhythmias of various kinds, including atrial fibrillation. Tachyarrhythmias are experienced by the patient as palpitations. A strong association between atrial tachyarrhythmias and systemic embolism has been demonstrated [34]. In addition to control of bradycardiac symptoms, another goal of pacing with the sick sinus syndrome is to prevent tachyarrhythmias. This can be achieved in two ways: (1) maintenance of atrial rate can prevent escape tachycardias, or (2) antibradycardic pacing can permit administration of antiarrhythmic agents that otherwise would not be tolerated.

From the foregoing it should be evident that atrial pacing is preferred for patients with the sick sinus syndrome. Nevertheless, it may be necessary to provide dual chamber pacing if any significant AV block exists or if antiarrhythmic drugs are used that might impair AV conduction. Thus the atrial demand mode, AAI, is chosen, with a back-up dual chamber mode (DDD) when necessary. Some patients, perhaps 5%–10%, display a severe inability to raise sinus rate to 100 bpm with exertion. New rate responsive modes of pacing by means of some sensor (see above) should then be considered, including AAIR or DDDR. These are now undergoing clinical testing. Reports of reductions in the incidence of heart failure, atrial arrhythmias, systemic embolism and mortality using atrial (or dual chamber) pacing as opposed to ventricular pacing have appeared [35, 36]. With ventricular pacing, there is no such reduction in mortality [37]. While these reports are encouraging, the place of atrial pacing in patients with sick sinus syndrome is not yet clear. It is sufficient to state that ventricular pacing alone is undesirable. This is because not only are the atria not paced, but also retrograde stimulation of the atria through the normal AV conduction system during the atrial vulnerable period may induce atrial tachyarrhythmias. Compounding this may be the adverse haemodynamic effects of retrograde atrial stimulation, which presents clinically as pacemaker syndrome (see above).

## Carotid Sinus Syndrome

Disordered heart rate control and bradycardia due to autonomic dysfunction, the carotid sinus syndrome, is of unknown aetiology. The diagnosis is made by 5 s of carotid sinus massage producing asystole lasting longer than 3 s in patients who have a history of syncope but in whom other causes for syncope have been excluded. It requires dual chamber stimulation for optimal haemodynamic benefit [38]. A minority (5%) of patients will remain symptomatic due to vasodepression in spite of pacing. There is a strong male predisposition and the average age of presentation is 70 years. Pacing does not prolong life and the 5-year survival rate is approximately 60% [39].

## Vasovagal Syndrome

Elderly patients who present with cardiac syncope, but in whom no aetiological abnormality is detected, have in the past been left undiagnosed and considered to have syncope of unknown origin or vasovagal syndrome. While emphasis has been placed on investigation of ventricular tachyarrhythmias as the cause for syncope in these patients, several recent reports indicate that 60° head-up tilt testing can induce vasovagal syncope in susceptible patients after about 25 min of tilt [14, 40]. Syncope is produced by bradycardia with hypotension in 80% of these, and hypotension without bradycardia (vasodepressor response) in the remainder [41]. Bradycardia patients have been markedly improved by dual chamber cardiac pacing [41]. Therapy for vasodepressor vasovagal syndrome is under investigation. Cutaneously administered scopolamine has been reported to be of benefit [40]. Vasovagal syndrome appears to have low mortality with or without pacing, but morbidity is considerable with injuries sustained in falls due to syncope in patients who are not paced.

## Pacemaker Implantation

Pacemakers are now almost exclusively implanted using local anaesthesia and a transvenous approach for the lead(s). The procedure is rapid: 30–60 min for a single chamber unit and 60–90 min for a dual chamber system. Moreover, the procedure has very few complications. Lead dislodgement is the most important complication and occurs in less than 1% of patients with ventricular leads [42] and in less than 2.5% of patients with atrial leads [43].

## Pacemaker Clinic

Patients require regular observation (every 6–12 months), not only to assess their clinical status but also to confirm pacemaker function and to check for battery depletion. Lithium batteries have predictable discharge characteristics, which provide early warning of impending power source depletion and permit elective pulse generator replacement. Battery lifetimes of 6–8 years can be anticipated.

## Late Complications

The pacemaker syndrome with VVI pacing was mentioned above. Pulse generator ulceration remains a problem although the reduction in the size and weight of pulse generators has lowered its incidence. Pulse generator ulceration presents initially as painless redness of the skin over a prominent part of the unit, which then often proceeds to ulceration. Infection does not become a part of this process until the skin breaks down. Relocation of the pulse generator at an early stage is the best treatment.

The environment both inside and outside the hospital presents potential hazards for patients with pacemakers. In pratice these hazards are minimal. Most daily activities, even those performed with or in the presence of household electronic devices, can be considered safe. As a general recommendation, surgical diathermy should not be undertaken unless pulse generator sensing function has been disabled either by use of a magnet or with programming. Lithotripsy and magnetic resonance imaging should not be undertaken without consultation with the implanting centre. The risks of these environmental hazards can be reduced with bipolar lead configurations (both electrodes in the heart) as opposed to unipolar lead systems (one electrode in the heart, the other being the metal can of the pulse generator).

## Prognosis of Pacemaker Patients

Age alone should not affect the decision to implant a pacemaker. One large study has shown that of all paced patients, females in their seventh or eighth decade have the best prognosis [44]. Conversely, patients for whom the best results might be anticipated, males in their fifth or sixth decade, fare poorly [45]. This would appear to be due to other complications of coronary artery disease.

## References


1 Elmquist R, Senning A (1959) An implantable pacemaker for the heart. In: Smyth CN (ed) Medical electronics. Proceedings of the 2nd International Conference on Medical Electronics. Illife, London, p 253

2 Bernstein AD, Camm AJ, Fletcher RD, Gold RD, Rickards AF, Smyth NPD, Spielman SR, Sutton R (1987) The NASPE*/BPEG Generic pacemaker code for antibradyarrhythmia and adaptive-rate pacing and antitachyarrhythmia devices. PACE 10:794–799

3 Nathan DA, Center S, Wu CY, Keller W (1963) An implantable synchronous pacemaker for the long term correction of complete heart block. Am J Cardiol 11:362–367

4 Rickards AF, Norman J (1981) Relation between QT interval and heart rate. New design of a physiologically adaptive cardiac pacemakeer. Br Heart J 45:56

5 Andersen C, Madsen GM (1990) Rate-responsive pacemakers and anaesthesia. A consideration of possible implications. Anaesthesia 45:472–476

6 Sutton R (1990) DDDR pacing. PACE 13:385–387

7 Kruse I, Arnman K, Conradson TB, Ryden L (1981) A comparison of the acute and long term haemodynamic effects of ventricular inhibited and atrial synchronous ventricular inhibited pacing. Circulation 65:846–855

8 Sutton R, Perrins EJ, Morley CA, Chan SL (1983) Sustained improvement in exercise tolerance following physiological cardiac pacing. Eur Heart J 4:781–786

9 Perrins EJ, Morley CA, Chan SL, Sutton R (1983) Randomised controlled trial of physiological and ventricular pacing. Br Heart J 50:112–117

10 Rankin I, Lindemans F (1985) Clinical evaluation of the Medtronic Activitrax single chamber rate variable implantable pulse generator. Medtronic Clinical Department, Research and Support Centre, Kerkrade

11 Benditt DG, Mianulli M, Fetter J, Benson DW, Dunningan A, Molina E, Gormick CC, Almquist A (1987) Single chamber cardiac pacing with activity-initiated chronotropic response: evaluation by cardiopulmonary exercise testing. Circulation 75:184–192

12 Lau CP, Rushby J, Leigh-Jones M, Tam CWF, Poloniecki J, Ingram A, Sutton R, Camm AJ (1989) Symptomatology and quality of life for patients with rate responsive pacemakers: a double-blind cross-over study. Clin Cardiol 12:505–512

13 Morley C, Sutton R (1984) Carotid sinus syndrome: Editorial Review. Int J Cardiol 6:287–293

14 Kenny RA, Ingram A, Bayliss J, Sutton R (1986) Head-up tilt: a useful test for investigating unexplained syncope. Lancet i:1352–1355

15 Kenny RA, Sutton R (1986) Pacemaker syndrome. Br Med J 293:902–903

16 Wong CK, Lauf CP, Cheng CH, Leung WH, Pun KK, Nicholls MG (1990) Delayed decline in plasma atrial natriuretic peptide levels after an abrupt reduction in atrial pressures: observation in patients with dual-chamber pacing. Am Heart J 120:882–885

17 Vardas PE, Travill CM, Williams TDM, Ingram AM, Lightman SL, Sutton R (1988) Effect of dual chamber pacing on raised plasma atrial natriuretic peptide concentrations in complete atrioventricular block. Br Med J 269:94

18 Travill CM, Williams TDM, Vardas P, Ingram A, Theodorakis G, Ahmed R, Chalmers J,

Lightman S, Sutton R (1989) Hypotension in pacemaker syndrome is associated with marked atrial natriuretic peptide release (ANP). PACE 12:1182.
19 Travill CM, Vardas P, Williams TDM, Ingram A, Lightman SL, Sutton R (1988) Atrial natriuretic peptide in different modes of cardiac pacing. New Trends Arrhythmias 4:789–793
20 Dhingra RC, Wyndham C, Bauernfeind R, Swiryn S, Deedwania PC, Smith T, Denes P, Rosen KM (1979) Significance of block distal to the His bundle induced by atrial pacing in patients with chronic bifasicular block. Circulation 60:1455
21 Saoudi N, Berland J, Hocq R, Cave D, Cribier A, Letac B (1986) Comparison des effets de l'ajmaline et de la procainamide dans le diagnostic du block auriculo-ventriculaire paroxystique. Ann Cardiol Angeiol (Paris) 36:13–17
22 Vardas P, Travill C, Bayliss J, Williams T, Sutton R (1987) Intravenous administration of flecainide as a stress test for syncopal patients with normal electrophysiology. PACE 10:A 514
23 Johansson BW (1966) Complete heart block. Acta Med Scand 180 [Suppl 451]:1–127
24 Fisher JD, Furman S, Escher DJW (1982) Pacing in the sick sinus syndrome. Profile and prognosis. In: Feruglio G (ed) Cardiac pacing, electrophysiology and pacemaker technology. Piccin, Padova, pp 519–520
25 Alpert MA, Curtis JJ, Sanfelippo JF, Flaker GC, Walls JT, Mukerji V, Villarreal D, Katti SK, Madigan NP, Krol RB (1986) Comparative survival after permanent ventricular and dual chamber pacing for patients with chronic high degree atrioventricular block with and without preexistent congestive heart failure. J Am Coll Cardiol 7:529–532
26 Davies MJ (1971) The pathology of the conducting tissue of the heart. Butterworth, London
27 Steinbeck G (1986) Diagnostische Elektrostimulation. In: Lüderitz B (ed) Herzschrittmacher. Therapie und Diagnostik kardialer Rhythmusstörungen. Springer, Berlin Heidelberg New York, pp 51–90
28 Michaelson J, Engle MA (1973) Congenital complete heart block: an international study of the natural history. Cardiovasc Clin 4:85–101
29 Davies MJ, Pomerance A (1972) Pathology of atrial fibrillation in man. Br Heart J 34:520–525
30 Abdon NJ (1981) Frequency and distribution of long term ECG recorded cardiac arrhythmias in an elderly population. Acta Med Scand 209:175–183
31 Freye RL, Collins JJ, De Sanctis RW, Dodge HT, Dreifus LS, Fisch C, Geths LS, Gillette PC, Parsonnet V, Reeves J, Weinberg SL (1984) Guidelines for permanent cardiac pacemaker implantation, May 1984. A report of the joint American College of Cardiology/-American Heart Association task force on assessment of cardiovascular procedures. Circulation 70:331 A–339 A
32 Narula OS, Samet P, Javier RP (1972) Significance of the sinus node recovery time. Circulation 45:140
33 Jose AD (1966) Effect of combined sympathetic and parasympathetic blockade on heart and cardiac function in man. Am J Cardiol 18:476–478
34 Fairfax AJ, Lambert CD, Leatham A (1976) Systemic embolism in chronic sino-atrial disorder. N Engl J Med 295:190
35 Sutton R, Kenny RA (1986) The natural history of sick sinus syndrome. PACE 9:110–114
36 Alpert MA, Curtis JJ, Sanfelippo JF, Flaker GC, Walls JT, Mukerji V, Villarreal D, Katti SK, Madigan NP, Morgan RJ (1987) Comparative survival following permanent ventricular and dual chamber pacing for patients with chronic symptomatic sinus node dysfunction with and without congestive heart failure. Am Heart J 113:958–965
37 Shaw DB, Holman RR, Gowers JI (1980) Survival in sino-atrial disorder (sick sinus syndrome). Br Med J 21:139–142
38 Morley CA, Perrins EJ, Sutton R (1982) Carotid sinus syncope treated by pacing. Analysis of persistant symptoms and role of atrioventricular sequential pacing. Br Heart J 47:411–418
39 Sutton R, Ahmed R, Ingram A (1989) 12 year experience of pacing in carotid sinus syndrome. PACE 12:1153
40 Abi-Samra F, Maloney JD, Fouad-Tarazi FM, Castle LW (1988) The usefulness of head-up

tilt testing and hemodynamic investigations in the workup of syncope of unknown origin. PACE 11:1202–1214
41 Fitzpatrick A, Sutton R (1989) Tilting towards a diagnosis – head-up tilt in the malignant vasovagal syndrome. Lancet i:658–660
42 Perrins EJ, Sutton R, Kalebic B, Richards LR, Morley CA, Terpstra B (1980) Modern atrial and ventricular leads for permanent cardiac pacing. Br Heart J 46:96–201
43 Kenny RA, Ingram A, Perrins EJ, Morley CA, Canepa-Anson R, Sutton R (1985) Unipolar and bipolar atrial leads – a six year experience. PACE 8:A 82
44 Ginks W, Siddons H, Leatham A (1979) Prognosis of patients paced for chronic atrioventricular block. Br Heart J 41:633–636
45 Ginks W, Sutton R, Siddons H, Leatham A (1980) Unsuspected coronary artery disease as a cause of chronic atrioventricular block in middle age. Br Heart J 44:699–702

# Rate-Responsive Cardiac Pacing

A. G. Hedman

During the past three decades cardiac pacing has made tremendous progress, which has enabled physicians to gradually increase the therapeutic ambition levels. While the initial goal was merely to keep patients with Adams-Stokes syndrome due to third degree atrioventricular (AV) block alive, pacing indications were expanded to include patients with symptomatic bradycardia due to sinus node dysfunction. With the development of atrial triggered ventricular pacing (VAT), it has become possible to preserve physiologic cardiovascular function to a much greater extent. The present interest in perceived well-being or issues relating to quality of life in pacemaker patients is a fine tribute to the advances made in cardiac pacing. Recently, modern pacemaker technology has permitted us to extend the benefits of ventricular rate variability to patients unsuitable for an atrial triggered system; we have thereby been able to meet the special needs of our patients, thus improving their quality of life — in other words, their perceived general well-being.

Although it is probably impossible to define "well-being", we can identify a number of factors which influence the quality of life. Apart from obvious social, economic or political factors beyond the control of the physician who implants pacemakers and manages patients with pacemakers, some medical determinants may be listed (Table 1). An adequate ventricular rate response is obviously important to achieve optimal well-being. But, is the ventricular rate the only important determinant or is AV synchrony also important? In the following, a number of controlled studies of various rate-responsive pacing systems are reviewed. All have in common a comparison of one rate-responsive mode to fixed-rate ventricular inhibited pacing (VVI), and all include an assessment of symptoms and/or patient preference for either pacing mode.

**Table 1.** Medical determinants of patient well-being

1. The patient should be asymptomatic
2. Physical capacities should be preserved
3. The patient should respond normally to mental stress
4. Both the doctor and the patient should have full confidence in the pacing system

## Assessment of Well-being

Since well-being is strictly a subjective phenomenon which incorporates many factors in a person's life, there can be no really objective measurements of patient well-being or quality of life. Even persons with quite severe physical disability may express a high degree of perceived well-being. For example, in a survey of a group of patients with very high spinal cord injury and ventilator dependence, 64% rated their quality of life as either excellent or good [1]. Only 10% rated their quality of life as poor or very poor.

The results of symptom-limited exercise tolerance tests and mental stress tests in patients with cardiovascular disease may well reflect functional capacity, but are by no means synonymous with perceived well-being. Nevertheless, functional capacity is of great importance to estimates of quality of life since perceived well-being is unlikely to be optimal if cardiovascular function is impaired.

The assessment of perceived well-being might be made by using symptom diaries kept by the patients and by specific questionnaires. Various psychological general indices of well-being have been developed and may be useful. When studying whether one pacing mode or type of pacemaker is superior to another, probably the best method is to compare pacing modes in a controlled study, preferably one with a double-blind, randomized, cross-over within-patient design. Such a study design might include objective measurement of exercise tolerance and evaluation of symptoms, so that patient preference for one of the modes can be determined without bias.

## Relationship Between Ventricular Rate and Exercise Capacity

Several controlled studies have demonstrated an improvement in physical capacity when the ventricular rate is allowed to increase with exercise by means of a rate-responsive pacing system. A review of the studies which compare VVI to one of a number of rate-responsive modes shows a remarkable correlation ($r = 0.92$; $P < 0.001$) between an increase in rate and improved exercise capacity [2]. This correlation is independent of the type of rate-responsive system used.

Pehrsson studied the influence of heart rate and AV synchronization on physical working capacity [3]. In this study, patients performed three exercise tests. For the first two tests, the ventricular endocardial lead was connected to an external pacemaker, which permitted manual alteration of the ventricular pacing rate. One of these two tests was performed with VVI pacing at 70 bpm. With the other, the ventricular rate was manually increased to approximately match the recorded atrial rate, but the ventricles were not synchronized with the atria. The third test was performed with VAT pacing. The working capacity was significantly higher with both atrial-matched ventricular and VAT pacing compared to VVI pacing. There was, however, no significant difference between atrial-matched ventricular and VAT pacing. Thus, existing data indicate that the ventricular rate is a more important determinant of exercise tolerance than AV synchrony per se.[1]

## Atrial-Triggered Versus VVI Pacing

Two controlled studies have compared perceived well-being during physiological (VDD or DDD modes: see Atlee, page 139, Table 1) and VVI pacing. The first double-blind, randomized, cross-over study was published by Perrins and co-workers in 1983 [4]. They found a 27% increase in exercise capacity ($p < 0.01$) with the physiological mode. Their patients were asked to report symptoms and score their general well-being during the two study periods. The subjective sensation of well-being was significantly improved during physiological pacing ($p < 0.01$). Patient preference for one or the other mode for pacing was not investigated in this study.

These early results were supported by those subsequently published by Kristensson et al. [5]. In 44 patients, the average increase in maximum heart rate with VDD pacing was 63% ($p < 0.001$), with a 14% improvement in exercise tolerance ($p < 0.01$). Patients reported more symptoms with VVI pacing, and their subjective impression of physical capacity was significantly ($p < 0.001$) in favor of VDD pacing. Twenty-nine of 44 patients (66%) preferred VDD pacing ($p < 0.001$), 20% had no preference, and 14% preferred VVI pacing. Finally, three of the five patients programmed to the VVI mode after termination of the study later requested reprogramming to VDD due to a perceived sense of diminished well-being.

## Single Chamber Rate-Responsive Versus VVI Pacing

### *Activity Sensor*

Smedgard and co-workers [6] studied an activity-sensing pacemaker system using a similar design to the above-mentioned study by Kristensson et al. [5]. Activity sensing by the pacemaker sensor was greater during treadmill than bicycle exercise since walking causes more body vibrations than pedalling a bicycle. The maximum rate was 112 bpm versus 97 bpm, respectively, corresponding to an improvement in exercise capacity by 19% ($p < 0.01$) on the treadmill and 7% ($p < 0.01$) during bicycle exercise. The score for subjective symptoms did not differ between the two pacing modes. Nevertheless, 13/15 patients preferred the rate-responsive (vs non-rate-responsive) period, mainly due to less dyspnea and tiredness. Two patients did not express

◀

[1]While existing data for conscious subjects may indicate that ventricular rate is a more important determinant of exercise tolerance than is proper AV synchrony, this may or may not apply to unconscious (anesthetized) patients, especially those with presumed impairment of ventricular diastolic function. Unpublished observations (J.L.A.) of the hemodynamic effects of transesophageal indirect atrial pacing (TAP) in anesthetized patients with hypertensive or ischemic cardiomyopathy (seven patients to date) indicate that both heart rate and preserved atrial transport are at least equally important mechanisms for augmentation of myocardial performance. In fact, preserved atrial transport with TAP may be more important than rate augmentation for improving cardiac performance in these same patients with AV junctional rhythm or during ventricular asynchronous pacing. These impressions are based on direct measurements of systemic and pulmonary artery pressures, thermal dilution cardiac output determinations, and derived indices of cardiac performance in these same patients.

any preference. An earlier study by Humen and co-workers [7] produced very similar results regarding maximum rate and exercise tolerance, but perceived well-being or patient preference was not investigated in that study.

## Evoked QT Interval Sensor

In a double-blind, randomized, cross-over study of 19 patients, Hedman and Nordlander found a 47% increase ($p < 0.001$) in maximum heart rate, corresponding to a 9% improvement ($p < 0.01$) in exercise tolerance, during QT-sensing pacing [8]. These findings were similar to the results of an earlier open study by Hedman and co-workers [9]. In the controlled study, the patients were asked to record episodes of chest pain, dyspnea, dizziness, or palpitations with both pacing modes. As in the study of the activity-sensing pacemaker by Smedgard and co-workers [6], there was no significant difference in number of symptom episodes between the modes. The patients rated their general well-being significantly higher with QT pacing ($p < 0.05$). Eleven of 19 patients preferred the rate-responsive mode, five had no preference, and two patients preferred the VVI pacing — one of the latter due to worsening of angina pectoris with QT pacing. The preference for the rate-responsive mode was statistically significant ($p < 0.05$).

## Comparison of Different Rate-Responsive System

To date, there are few studies which compare the effects of different single-chamber, rate-responsive pacing systems on perceived well-being of patients. Kay et al. have published a study of 22 patients, 10 with activity-sensing and 12 with minute-ventilation sensing system [10]. Physical performance and well-being were investigated using the same protocol for both groups. There were no differences between the two pacing systems in improvement in physical function or quality of life parameters. A weakness of this study is the comparison of two different small populations. Obviously more data are needed in this area, and the development of multi-sensor pacemakers will permit such studies.

## Atrial-Triggered Versus Ventricular Rate-Responsive Pacing

The recent development of AV universal pacemakers (DDD) which are rate responsive (DDDR) permits within-patient comparisons of DDD and VVIR [11]. A study by Sulke et al. [12], at present available only in abstract form, included 22 patients with second or third degree atrioventricular block, 17 of whom also had sinus node incompetence, and seven with retrograde AV (VA) conduction. All had activity-sensing DDDR generators implanted. The study design was randomized, double-blind, and cross-over, and comprised four test periods, each 4 weeks long. The generators were programmed to DDD, DDDR, DDIR, and VVIR, respectively. Evaluation included a subjective (patient) assessment, treadmill exercise testing, standardized daily activities, and echocardiography.

Objective exercise tolerance, i.e., time on the treadmill, was similar in all modes, but was worse subjectively in the VVIR mode than in all dual chamber modes ($p > 0.05$). Cardiac output was lower with VVIR at rest, but similar with all modes at 120 bpm. Regarding preference, five patients demanded early cross-over, all from the VVIR mode. Thirteen patients preferred DDDR, four preferred DDIR, four preferred any dual chamber pacing mode, and one patient with poor left ventricular function preferred VVIR. Perceived well-being was worse with VVIR compared to DDD ($p < 0.05$) or DDDR ($p < 0.01$) pacing. No significant difference was found between VVIR and DDIR.

Hummel et al. studied patients with sinus node disease and found that rate-responsive DDD was better tolerated than rate-responsive VVI [13]. Interestingly, in a small single-blind, cross-over study of eight patients with AV block without sinus node incompetence, Bubien and Kay found that quality of life parameters and exercise tolerance were similar with DDD and VVIR, but that with respect to perceived well-being, patients still preferred the DDD mode [14]. These results suggest that patients might be aware of some subtle differences, possibly related to the preservation of atrial function at rest.

## Conclusions

Available controlled studies all show that the type of pacing system does indeed influence perceived well-being by patients. Rate-adaptive systems consistently provide increased exercise tolerance when compared to fixed-rate ventricular pacing, seemingly regardless of the type of sensor used to achieve rate-responsive pacing. Furthermore, most patients report an improved sense of well-being with a rate-responsive system and usually express a preference for the more physiological pacing mode. Finally, this review suggests that pacemaker-dependent patients should be offered a rate-responsive system, but there is still insufficient evidence to recommend any particular type of sensor for a majority of patients. In certain patients, e.g., those with a combination of atrioventricular block and sinus node disease, there is evidence that a dual-chamber system (DDD or DDDR, as applicable) might be more favorable than a rate-responsive VVI system.

## References


1 Whiteneck GG, Carter RE, Charlifue SW et al. (1985) A collaborative study of high quadriplegia. Craig Hospital, Englewood
2 Nordlander R, Hedman A, Pehrsson SK (1989) Rate responsive pacing and exercise capacity – a comment. PACE 12:749–751
3 Pehrsson SK (1983) Influence of heart rate and atrioventricular synchronization on maximal work tolerance in patients treated with artificial pacemakers. Acta Med Scand 214:311–315
4 Perrins EJ, Morley CA, Chan SL, Sutton R (1983) Randomized clinical trial of physiological and ventricular pacing. Br Heart J 50:112–117
5 Kristensson BE, Arnman K, Smedgard P, Ryden L (1985) Physiological versus single-rate ventricular pacing: a double-blind cross-over study. PACE 8:73–84
6 Smedgard P, Kristensson BE, Kruse I, Ryden L (1987) Rate responsive pacing by means of activity sensing versus single rate ventricular pacing. PACE 10:902–915

7 Humen DP, Kostuk WJ, Klein GJ (1985) Activity-sensing, rate responsive pacing: improvement in myocardial performance with exercise. PACE 8:52–59
8 Hedman A, Nordlander R (1989) QT sensing rate responsive pacing compared to fixed rate ventricular pacing – a controlled clinical study. PACE 12:374–385
9 Hedman A, Nordlander R, Pehrsson SK, Astrom H (1986) Clinical experience with rate responsive pacing by the evoked QT. Stimucœur 14:22–26
10 Kay GN, Bubien RS, Karst GL (1989) Metabolic versus activity sensors for rate-adaptive pacing; a prospective comparison utilizing quality of life measurements. PACE 12:641 (abstract)
11 Sutton R (1990) DDDR pacing. PACE 13:385–387
12 Sulke N, Dritsas A, Chambers J et al. (1990) A randomized cross-over study of four rate responsive pacing modes. PACE 13:534 (abstract)
13 Hummel J, Barr E, Hanich R, McElroy B, Brinker J (1990) DDDR pacing is better tolerated than VVIR in patients with sinus node disease. PACE 13:504 (abstract)
14 Bubien RS, Kay GN (1990) A randomized comparison of quality of life and exercise capacity with DDD and VVIR pacing modes. PACE 13:524 (abstract)

# Pacemakers in Children

J. I. STEIN, D. DACAR, H. METZLER, P. SOVINZ*, AND A. BEITZKE

## Introduction

Both historical reports of stimulating the heart by shocking it through the chest in the 18th century and the first attempts to pace the heart percutaneously in 1932 dealt with children [1]. Despite this, permanent pacemaker implantations in children, though increasing in number, still account for only a small percentage of implanted pacemaker systems. Ninety percent of patients with pacemakers are older than 60 years.

Advances in pacemaker technology and implantation techniques first benefited the adult population. Nevertheless, since the first reports of successful permanent pacing in children in the 1960s, more reliable pacing systems have been developed for this age group [2–14]. The complication rate for pacing in the pediatric age group is still quite high, and often due to physiological changes that occur with protracted pacing. Multiple reoperations are required for battery replacement, and also for revision of leads and replacement of pulse generators. Children with pacemakers also face various psychological and social problems [15, 16].

An update on the rapid technical developments in this field has recently been provided by Kugler [16]. Here we describe our 17 years experience with permanent cardiac pacing in the pediatric age group.

## Patient Population

Between 1973 and 1990, permanent cardiac pacemaker systems were implanted in 53 patients (32 male, 21 female) aged 1 day to 18 years (mean 5.5 ± 4.3 years). There were 16 children with congenital conduction disturbances who required pacing at a mean age of 7 ± 5.3 years (1 day to 18 years). In the remaining 37 patients, pacemaker therapy became necessary following corrective surgery for congenital heart disease at a mean age of 4.8 ± 3.7 years (2 months to 12.8 years). The age distribution of patients is shown in Fig. 1. There were six babies weighing less than 10 kg, including two newborns weighing 2 kg and 3.2 kg, respectively.

The time interval between cardiac surgery and pacemaker implantation ranged from intraoperative implantation (three patients) to 10.7 years (0.94 ± 2.15 years). In 28 of the 37 patients (75%) the pacemaker was implanted within 1 month postoperatively; in another two it was implanted within 1 year, in five within 5 years, and in only two after more than 5 years (5.3 and 10.7 years).

---

*Sponsored by a grant from Verein Hilfe für das herzkranke Kind, Graz, Austria

The most common diagnostic categories for the underlying cardiac malformation of postoperative patients were transposition of the great arteries and atrioventricular and ventricular septal defects. Associated cardiac lesions were present in 8 of the 16 children with congenital conduction disturbances (Table 1).

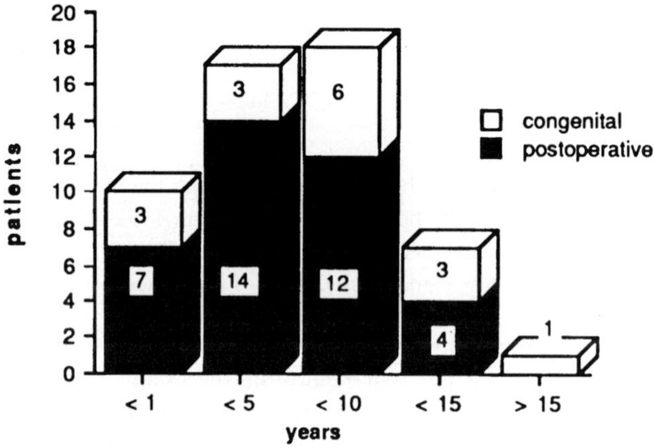


**Figure 1.** Patient age distribution at time of initial pacemaker implantation for congenital conduction disturbances (*open bars*) or conduction defects following corrective surgery for congenital heart disease (*shaded bars*)

**Table 1.** Associated (surgical) or underlying (congenital block) congenital malformations in patients with pacemakers

| Diagnosis | Surgical (*n*) | Congenital block (*n*) |
|---|---|---|
| R-TGA (± VSD, PST) | 8 | |
| L-TGA (± VSD, PST) | 4 | 1 |
| TOF (DORV) | 5 | |
| VSD | 8 | |
| AVSD | 6 | 1 |
| ASD | 1 | 1 |
| cor triatriatum | 1 | |
| MVR | 3 | |
| AVR | 1 | |
| PST | | 2 |
| PDA | | 1 |
| TA, VSD, PST | | 1 |
| DILV, Coa | | 1 |
| | 37 | 8 |

TGA, transposition of the great arteries; VSD, ventricular septal defect; PST pulmonary valve stenosis; TOF tetralogy of Fallot; DORV, double outlet right ventricle, AVSD, atrioventricular septal defect; ASD, atrial septal defect; A (M) VR, aortic (mitral) valve replacement; PDA, patent ductus arteriosus; TA, tricuspid atresia; DILV, double inlet left ventricle; Coa, coarctation of the aorta

## Indications

*Complete atrioventricular block* was the most frequent indication (85% of patients) for pacing in our patient population (Table 2). It was of congenital origin in 15 children and occurred postoperatively in another 30. Six children had symptomatic *sick sinus syndrome*. Five patients developed it postoperatively: four patients 1 week and 3, 3.5, and 10.7 years after Rastelli, Mustard, and Senning (two patients) type repair of transposition of the great arteries, and one patient 2.9 years after repair of tetralogy of Fallot. One patient had no associated cardiac anomaly but required pacing for sick sinus syndrome at the age of 10 years. Finally, in two patients, postoperative *bradyarrhythmia* of AV-junctional origin was the indication for pacing. In one patient, pacing was instituted 1 week after closure of a ventricular septal defect, and in the other 5.3 years following a Mustard operation.

## Implantation Technique

Initial pacer implantation was with epicardial screw-in leads in 41 patients (4.71 ± 4.15 years). The transvenous approach was chosen in the remaining 12 patients (8.35 ± 3.6 years). Multiprogrammable pulse generators were implanted in all patients (Table 3). Ventricular demand pacemakers (VVI) were implanted in most patients (75%) (Table 4) and the abdominal wall was the main implantation site.

**Table 2.** Underlying rhythm disturbance ($n = 53$)

| | Congenital disease | Surgical patients | Overall |
|---|---|---|---|
| Complete Atrioventricular block | 15 | 30 | 45 |
| Sick sinus syndrome | 1 | 5 | 6 |
| Bradyarrhythmia | – | 2 | 2 |
| | 16 | 37 | 53 |

**Table 3.** Types of initially implanted pulse generator systems (n = 53)

| Manufacturer | System | Number |
|---|---|---|
| Biotronics | Nomos | 3 |
| | Neos | 9 |
| | Mikros | 16 |
| | Kalos | 2 |
| Medtronics | Spectrax | 13 |
| | Activitrax | 7 |
| | Minix | 2 |
| | Synergist | 1 |

**Table 4.** Pacing modes and leads in the first implanted pacemaker system ($n = 53$)

| | No. | % |
|---|---|---|
| *Mode*[a] | | |
| VVI | 35 | 66 |
| VVI-R | 5 | 9 |
| DDD | 5 | 9 |
| DDD-R | 6 | 11 |
| AAI | 2 | 4 |
| *Leads* | | |
| Transvenous | 12 | 23 |
| Epimyocardial | 41 | 77 |

[a]For ICHD pacemaker identification codes for mode of pacing, see Atlee, page 139, Table 1

## Complications and Reoperations

The mean survival time for the first implanted pacemaker system was 3.3 ± 2.5 years, with a range of 1 month to 8 years. Twenty-three children (43%) required a total of 44 reoperations: 12 of these have had one reoperation, six have had two, three have had three, one has had five, and one has had six. Twelve reoperations were performed for problems with leads caused by growth (8), dislocation (1), erosion (2), or infection (1). In four patients the pulse generator was changed at the same time; in the remaining eight patients pulse generators were replaced at the subsequent operation.

Early pacing threshold rise was the indication for system replacement in four patients. The time between initial implantation and revision in these patients was 1, 2, 4, and 6 weeks. In one patient, infection at the implantation site in the abdominal wall was the reason for changing the pacing system. All these complications occurred in patients with epimyocardial screw-in leads.

Mean time of follow-up is 5.05 ± 4.33 years (3 months to 17 years). There were seven deaths during this follow-up period; none of them was related to pacing failure. Three patients in the postoperative group with associated Down's syndrome died because of pulmonary hypertension. One died due to low cardiac output syndrome 3 days after repair of an interrupted aortic arch and ventricular septal defect, another of right ventricular failure 6 years after a Mustard operation and 9 months after pacemaker implantation. Two deaths in pacemaker patients with congenital complete atrioventricular block occurred 1 week and 3 months after corrective surgery for the associated congenital heart disease.

## Discussion

Congenital or acquired (following intracardiac surgery) complete atrioventricular block is the most common indication for permanent pacemaker therapy in childhood [4, 6, 12–14, 16–19]. In the series reviewed by Ward [13] and Kugler [16], pacing for postoperative atrioventricular block constitutes the indication for pacing in between

56% and 61%, respectively, of all children with permanent pacemaker therapy. In the majority, pacing is required within 1 month after surgery.

Patients with congenital complete atrioventricular block, whether or not associated with cardiac anomalies, are known to be at high risk for developing symptoms of syncope or dizziness, or even experiencing sudden death [4, 11, 16]. Therefore, these patients must be followed closely with frequent 24- to 48-hour Holter-ECG monitoring, and considered for permanent pacing if symptoms occur or mean heart rate falls below 50 beats/min [16].

The overall incidence of complete atrioventricular block as the indication for permanent pacemaker therapy in our patient population was 85% – 57% postoperatively and 28% for congenital block. About 75% of patients who required pacing for acquired complete atrioventricular block did so by 1 month, whereas in only 2 of 16 with congenital atrioventricular block was pacemaker therapy necessary in the 1st week of life. These two newborns, weighing 2 and 3.2 kg, were in cardiac failure and had associated cardiac lesions.

There has been some discussion about intraoperative prophylactic pacemaker implantation [14, 16]. We, like others, do not recommend this approach, since improvement of the conduction disturbance and even restoration of normal sinus rhythm may occur during the first postoperative weeks [16]. We observed this in one of our three patients with intraoperative pacemaker implantation. Intraoperative mapping can further decrease the risk of unnecessary early pacemakeer implantation [13, 14, 20].

The second major indication for permanent pacing is *the sick sinus syndrome,* which usually develops later after surgery [6, 16]. In our cases, as well as in those reported in the literature, sinus node dysfunction is most likely to occur following intraatrial surgery. Possibly this is due to damage to the sinus node during Mustard, Senning, or Fontan type procedures, or closure of atrial septal defects [6, 16, 17]. Thus, the incidence of sick sinus syndrome is expected to increase with increasing length of follow-up. Sick sinus syndrome associated with tetralogy of Fallot, as occurred in one of our patients, is unusual but has been reported by other authors, too [13, 16].

The indications for pacemaker implantation are chiefly based on clinical symptoms; reference is also made to surface ECG findings and the results of continuous ECG monitoring either immediately postoperatively or later with ambulatory (Holter) ECG. Electrophysiological studies may be required for precise diagnosis in some patients [6, 13, 19].

Although improvement in lead technology has increased the number of transvenous implantations [3, 5, 12, 21, 22], even in neonates [23], transthoracically inserted epimyocardial screw-in leads are still used in the majority of pediatric patients [2, 6–8, 10, 11, 13, 14, 17]. The latter technique has advantages in infants, in whom the vessels may still be too small for a transvenous lead and there is no other place besides the abdominal wall for the pulse generator. This cosmetic aspect sometimes also plays a role in older children. In some patients with complex lesions and epicardial adhesions after previous surgery the transvenous approach may have advantages [5, 22, 24].

In all children requiring a pacemaker, the long-term need for pacing and later

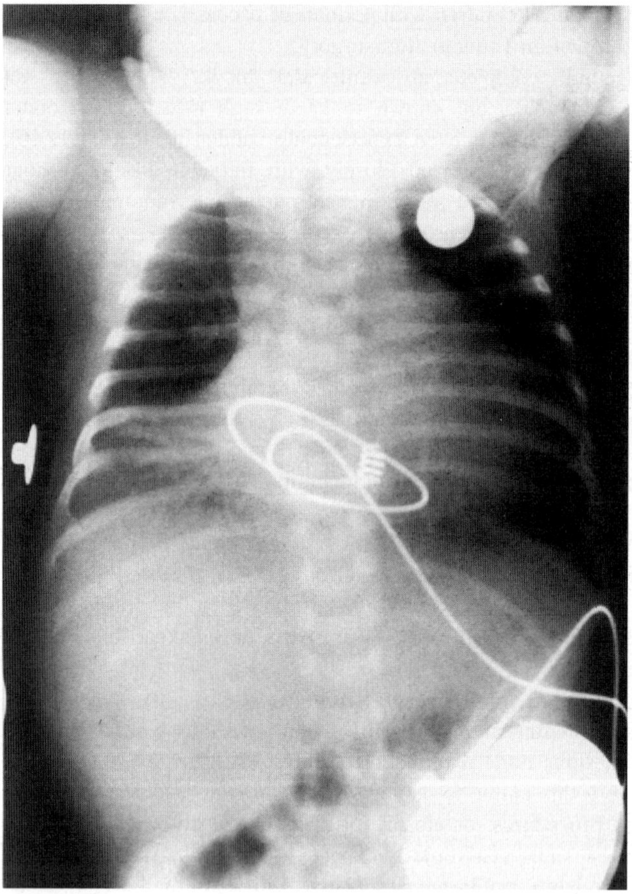

**Figure 2.** Chest x-ray of a 2-kg newborn with a Medtronic Minix generator implanted in the abdominal wall and an epimyocardial lead. Note the mismatch in size between the pulse generator and the patient

growth have to be kept in mind. To allow for growth, the first implanted lead must have some reserve length. A loop in the right atrium can accomplish this [12, 21, 23].

With the development of multiprogrammable generator systems of reduced size, almost all types of pacemaker systems are now available for use in children. Nevertheless, in neonates there can still be a mismatch of pulse generator and patient size (Fig. 2). Depending on the underlying electrophysiological disturbance, single or dual chamber pacing is possible, as well as fixed rate, rate adaptive, or inhibited sensing and pacing [6, 16, 18].

The general *Guidelines for Permanent Cardiac Pacemaker Implantation* provided by the Joint Task Force of the American College of Cardiology and The American Heart Association in 1984 [25] have recently been updated by Kugler [16] and revised by the Committee on Pacemaker Implantation in 1991 [26]. In young children with complete atrioventricular block and epimyocardial leads, rate adaptive VVI-R (VVI-R) pacing is currently the most commonly used mode since it permits increased exercise tolerance [16, 18]. In patients with sinus node dysfunction, single chamber, rate adaptive pacing (AAI-R or VVI-R) seems most advantageous. Rate adaptive dual chamber pacing (DDD-R) offers a new approach to pacing for older children with transvenous leads [16, 18].

There is still a considerable rate of complications requiring either lead or system replacement [2, 6, 9–11, 17]. Most of the complications are due to the special problem of growth and requirement for long-term pacing in pediatric patients. Another reason is the increase in pacing threshold which is especially likely to occur in patients who have undergone cardiac surgery and have pacing with epimyocardial leads [10]. In an attempt to reduce some of the complications, a new intrathoracic pulse generator implantation site has been proposed [27, 28].

No significant differences have been reported betweeen transvenous and epicardial leads with regard to longevity, although the overall performance of transvenous leads seems to be better [2, 6, 9, 10, 16, 18, 21, 24]. However, epimyocardial screw-in leads, especially if secured by a suture, seem to have a better performance with respect to pacing thresholds than epimyocardial stab-on leads [7]. The development of steroid-eluting lead systems may further improve lead performance [23].

The psychosocial response of children with cardiac pacemakers seems to be reasonably normal, since they can cope with the stress of their situation using denial and intellectualization [15]. For pacemaker follow-up in children, there are no special guidelines. The aim is to detect pacemaker system failure early, to achieve maximum benefit by programming the pulse generator to the most suitable mode for individual patients, and to maximize system longevity. For this, teamwork between the pediatric cardiologist and the implanting surgeon is essential.

Peri- and intraoperative management of children with pacemakers is different from that in adults. In all children pacemaker implantation should be performed under general anesthesia with controlled ventilation. If the transvenous approach is chosen, PEEP ventilation with 5–10 $cmH_2O$ should be applied. Concerning precautions to be taken for pacemaker exposure to electromagnetic interference (magnetic resonance imaging, computerized tomography, microwaves, or electrocautery), it is recommended that pacemakers be reprogrammed to asynchronous operation. If this is impractical or not feasible, then the implanting physician or clinic, or the pacemaker manufacturer, should be consulted as to appropriate alternative management.

## Summary

Permanent cardiac pacemaker therapy in childhood in most instances is for patients with complete atrioventricular block. In the majority of patients this occurs after surgery for congenital heart disease. Major problems faced with pacing in children are their small size, potential for growth, and life-long requirement for pacing. With advances in pacemaker technology, including the development of small, multiprogrammable pacing units and more reliable lead systems, many of these problems can be surmounted or at least minimized.

## References


1 Gamble WJ, Owens JP (1977) Pacemaker therapy for conduction defects in the pediatric population. In: Roberts N, Gelband H (eds) Cardiac arrhythmias in the neonate, infant and child. Appleton-Century-Crofts, New York, pp 469–525

2 Ector H, Dhooghe G, Daenen W, Stalpaert G, Hauwaert van der L, Geest De H (1985) Pacing in children. Br Heart J 53:541–546

3 Epstein ML, Knauf DG, Alexander JA (1986) Long-term follow-up of transvenous cardiac pacing in children. Am J Cardiol 57:889–890

4 Esscher E, Michaelsson M (1979) Assessment and management of complete heart block. In: Godman MJ, Marquis RM (eds) Heart disease in the newborn. Pediatric cardiologgy, vol 2 Churchill Livingstone, Edinburgh, pp 433–441

5 Gillette PC, Zeigler V, Bradham GB, Kinsella P (1988) Pediatric transvenous pacing: a concern for venous thrombosis? PACE 11:1935–1939

6 Goldmann BS, Williams WG, Hill T, Hesslein PS, McLaughlin PR, Trusler GA, Baird RJ (1985) Permanent cardiac pacing after open heart surgery: congenital heart disease. PACE 8:732–739

7 Kugler J, Monsour W, Blodgett C, Cheatham J, Gumbiner C, Hofschire P, Watson L, Fleming W (1988) Comparison of myoepicardial pacemaker leads: follow-up in 80 children, adolescents and young adults. PACE 11:2216–2222

8 McGrath LB, Gonzalez-Lavin L, Morse DP, Levett JM (1988) Pacemaker system failure and other events in children with surgically induced heart block. PACE 11:1182–1187

9 Serwer GA, Mericle JM (1987) Evaluation of pacemaker pulse generator and patient longevity in patients aged 1 day to 20 years. Am J Cardiol 59:824–827

10 Serwer GA, Mericle JM, Armstrong BE (1988) Epicardial ventricular electrode longevity in children. Am J Cardiol 61:104–106

11 Villain E, Seletti L, Kachaner J, Planche C, Sidi D, Bidois Le J (1989) Artificial cardiac stimulation in the newborn infant with complete congenital atrioventricular block. Study of 16 cases. Arch Mal Coeur 82:739–744

12 Walsh CA, McAlister HF, Andrews CA, Steeg CN, Eisenberg R, Furman S (1988) Pacemaker in children: a 21-year experience. PACE 11:1940–1944

13 Ward DE (1983) Permanent pacing in children. In: Anderson RH, Macartney FJ, Shinebourne EA, Tynan M (eds) Pediatric cardiology, vol 5 Churchill Livingstone, Edinburgh, pp 34–45

14 Ward DE, Signy M, Oldershaw P, Jones S, Shinebourne EA (1982) Cardiac pacing in children. Arch dis Child 57:514–520

15 Alpern D, Uzark K, Dick II M (1989) Psychosocial responses of children to cardiac pacemakers. J Pediatr 114:494–501

16 Kugler JD, Danford DA (1989) Pacemakers in children: an update. Am Heart J 117:665–679

17 Brüggemann G, Steil E, Barth H, Huth C, Apitz J (1988) Cardiac pacing in children. Klin Pädiatr 200:399–403

18 Karpawich PP, Perry BL, Farooki ZQ, Clapp SK, Jackson WL, Cicalese CA, Green EW (1986) Pacing in children and young adults with nonsurgical atrioventricular block: comparison of single-rate ventricular and dual-chamber modes. Am Heart J 13:316–321

19 Karpawich PP, Gillette PC, Carson A Jr, Hesslein PS, Porter CJ, McNamara DG (1981) Congenital complete atrioventricular block: clinical and electrophysiologic predictors of need for pacemaker insertion. Am J Cardiol 48:1098–1102

20 Lincoln C, Butler P, Logan-Sinclair R, Anderson RH (1979) A cardiac conduction monitor and probe for intraoperative identification of conduction tissue. Br Heart J 42:339–344

21 Iberer F, Tscheliessnigg W, Stenzl D, Dacar D, Rigler B, Mächler H, Kraft-Kinz J (1987) Seven years experience with growth-adapting electrodes for transvenous pacing in childhood. PACE 10:690–698

22 Ward DE, Jones S, Shinebourne EA (1987) Long-term transvenous pacing in children weighing ten kilograms or less. Int J Cardiol 15:112–115

23 Till JA, Jones S, Rowland E, Shinebourne EA, Ward DE (1989) Endocardial pacing in children: long term clinical experience with steroid eluting lead. III. World Congress of Pediatric Cardiology, Bangkok, 1989, p 178 (abstract)
24 Spotnitz HM 81990) Transvenous pacing in infants and children with congenital heart disease. Ann Thorac Surg 49:495–496
25 Frye RL, Collins JJ, DeSanctis RW, Dodge HT, Dreifus LS, Fisch C, Gettes LS, Gillette PC, Parsonnet V, Reeves J, Weinberg SL (1984) Guidelines for permanent cardiac pacemaker implantation. Circulation 70:331A–339A
26 Dreifus LS, Fisch C, Griffin JC, Gillette PC, Mason JW, Parsonnet V (1991) Guidelines of cardiac pacemakers and antiarrhythmia devices. JACC 18:1–13
27 Nikol S, Minale C, Engelhardt W, Messmer BJ (1990) New site for pacemaker generators in children. Eur J Cardiothorac Surg 4:342–344
28 Kiso I, Hirotani T, Maehara T, Yozu R, Umezu Y, Ishikura Y (1990) Intrathoracic pacemaker implantation in children. Kyobu Geka 43:280–282

# Implantable Cardioverter-Defibrillators

P. D. CHAPMAN

## Preoperative Considerations

Sudden cardiac death due to malignant ventricular arrhythmias is one of the nation's leading public health problems. An individual suffering such an event has only a 25% chance of survival [1]. Furthermore, patients suffering such an episode are at high risk for recurrent cardiac arrest. Through the pioneering efforts of Mirowski and colleagues [2], the implantable cardioverter-defibrillator (ICD) was conceived, developed, and successfully introduced as a treatment modality to prevent the malignant consequences of recurrent sustained ventricular tachyarrhythmias. The device continously monitors the cardiac rhythm and is capable of delivering a series of cardioverting or defibrillating shocks in an attempt to terminate ventricular tachycardia or fibrillation.

## Description and Functional Characteristics of the ICD

The only FDA-approved ICD device at present is manufactured by Cardiac Pacemakers, Inc. (St. Paul, MN). The titanium ICD pulse generator is much larger than a permanent pacemakers pulse generator. Its weight is 235 g and volume 145 ml (dimensions 10.1 cm x 7.6 cm x 2.0 cm) (Fig. 1). It is powered by two, lithium-silver vanadium pentoxide cells connected in series [3]. Because the device is bulky, it is not suitable for prepectoral implantation. Consequently, it is placed subcutaneously, typically in the left upper quadrant of the abdomen.

The pulse generator is connected to a lead system for sensing and defibrillation. The lead system is composed of two leads for defibrillation (Fig. 2). This may include a transvenous spring electrode paired with an epicardial patch electrode (spring-patch configuration) or, more commonly, two epicardial patch electrodes (patch-patch configuration). The patch-patch configuration is preferred because of lower defibrillation energy requirements and therefore a better safety margin [4]. The sensing leads for the ICD used for counting the heart rate may consist of either two epicardial screw-in electrodes or a transvenous bipolar electrode placed at the right ventricular apex.

In the active mode, the ICD device continuously monitors the cardiac rhythm. There are currently two possible sensing algorithms for arrhythmia detection: heart

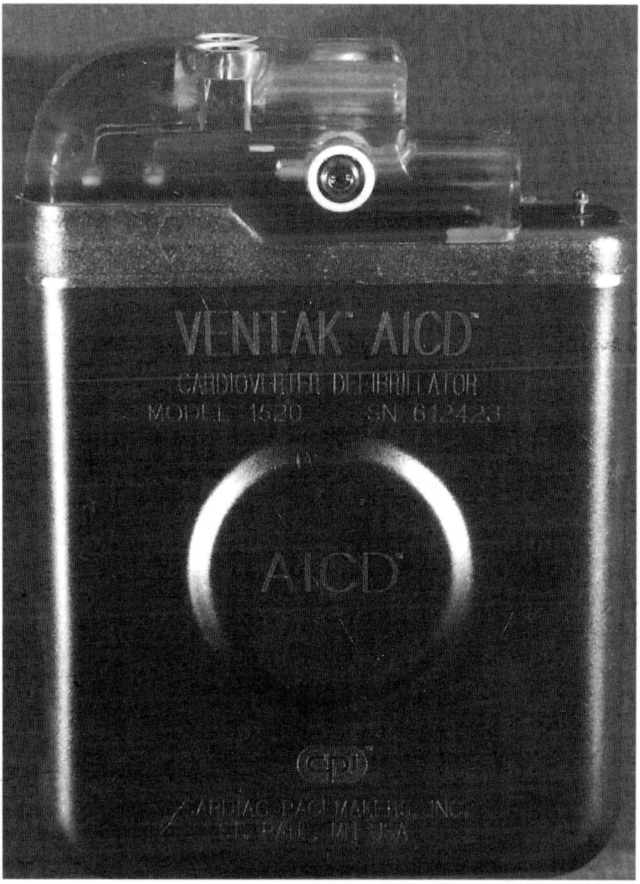


**Fig. 1.** Photograph of the automatic implantable cardioverter-defibrillator Ventak pulse generator

rate only and rate plus waveform analysis. Rate only devices will detect any heart rhythm faster than the programmable rate cutoff and cause the device to charge its capacitors and deliver a shock. The device requires 5–10s to "recognize" an arrhythmia and an additonal 10–20s to charge and deliver a shock.

Waveform analysis or probability density function is satisfied when the electrogram from the shocking leads has a shape that is more sinusoidal than normal sinus rhythm. This sinusoidal pattern would be typical of malignant ventricular arrhythmia. The potential advantage of this additional detection parameter is that it may decrease the likehood of detecting and treating narrow QRS supraventricular tachycardia.

After the device has delivered its first shock (programmable to 26 or 30J), it is capable of delivering up to four more shocks (30J each). Ten to 20s will elapse between shocks. After the full sequence of five shocks, the device requires a period of normal rhythm (approximately 35 s) before it can recycle and deliver another shock or series of shocks. The generator has an anticipated monitoring life of 4–5 years or will deliver 100–150 shocks.

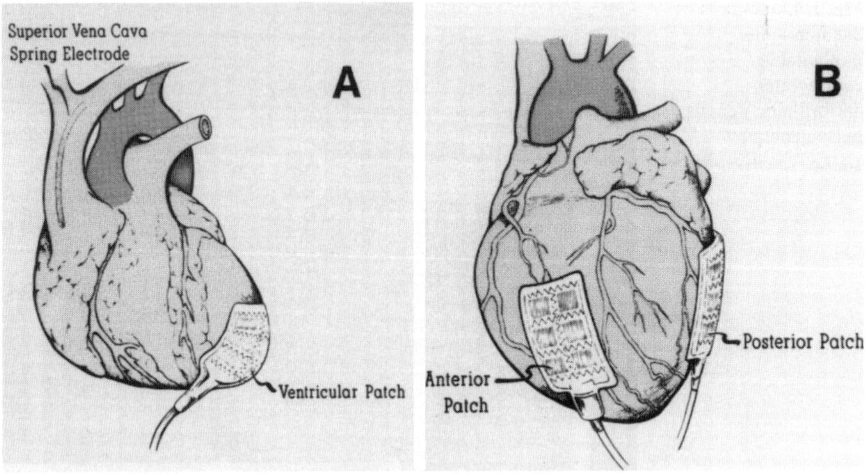


**Fig. 2 A, B.** Lead configurations for defibrillation with the ICD. *A* spring-patch configuration; *B* patch-patch configuration. See text for further discussion

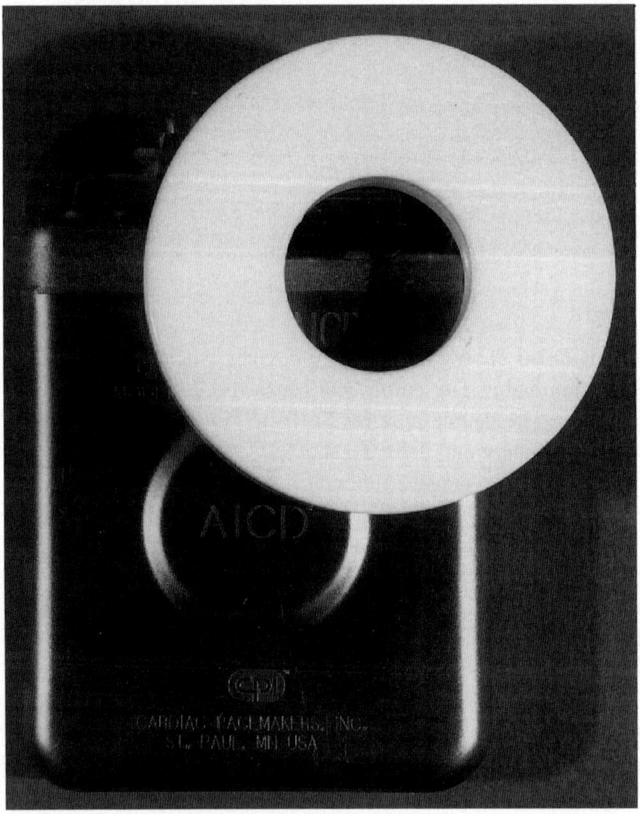


**Fig. 3.** Photograph demonstrating appropriate positioning of the toroid magnet to allow interaction with pulse generator. The magnet can activate/deactivate and divert shocks. See text for discussion

Interaction with and programming of the ICD device are performed with an external programmer with the programming wand placed over the pulse generator. Using this external device, the pulse generator can be activated/deactivated, the rate cutoff for detection can be programmed (110–200 beats per minute in 5 beat per minute increments), and the morphology component of the detection algorithm can be turned on or off. Additionally, first shock energy can be programmed to either 26 or 30J.

In addition to the programmer, one can use an external toroid (doughnut shaped) magnet to interact with the pulse generator. This magnet can activate/deactivate the device and can divert shocks from the patient to an internal resistance load. When the toroid magnet is positioned to interact with the generator [flat on the skin over the generator over the upper third of the device (Fig. 3)] audible tones will be heard. If the device is inactive, a continuous tone will be heard. Magnet application for approximately 30s will then activate the device and convert the continuous tone to QRS synchronous tones. Importantly, any time a magnet is interacting with the pulse generator, the ICD is inhibited from responding to any arrhythmias (it will not deliver a shock). This maneuver can be very useful if a patient (under closely monitored conditions) is receiving inappropriate shocks from the device (due to device malfunction or supraventricular arrhythmias at rates faster than the programmed rate cutoff for arrhythmia detection). In this situation, magnet application will divert further energy to the internal resistor and after 30 s will deactivate the pulse generator.

## Clinical Results of ICD Therapy

The ICD is approved for patients surviving a cardiac arrest associated with malignant ventricular arrhythmia (not due to acute myocardial infarction or reversible metabolic cause) and patients with sustained ventricular tachycardia not responsive to pharmacologic therapy [5].

Results of ICD therapy in these patient groups have been impressive, with a reported 5-year survival rate of 92% following impending sudden death [6]. Randomized comparison of drug therapy versus ICD therapy has not been performed but retrospective comparison with drug-related patients suggests clear superiority of the ICD. Tordjman-Fuchs et al. have reported a 1-year survival rate of 98% with the ICD, versus 71% in patients treated with antiarrhythmic drugs (patients treated prior to ICD availability) [7]. These impressive results have led some to conclude that ICD therapy is the treatment of choice for survivors of cardiac arrest unassociated with acute myocardial infarction [8].

## Anesthesia for ICD Implantation

The surgical procedure for ICD implantation requires entry into the thorax for installation of the patch electrode(s). Therefore, general anesthesia is required for the operation. Surgical approaches have included midline sternotomy (generally in patients undergoing concomitant cardiac surgery), anterior or lateral thoracotomy, and subxiphoid thoracotomy.

Appropriate monitoring of cardiac rhythm, arterial blood pressure, and central venous pressure should be established prior to induction of general anesthesia. A pulmonary artery catheter may be indicated in patients with compromised ventricular function. The anesthetic agents and technique will depend upon patient characteristics and underlying disease and whether additonal cardiac surgery is planned or performed. In patients with borderline cardiac compensation, fluid administration should be judicious.

It is important ro realize that the defibrillation energy requirements determined at the time of implantation in the anesthetized patient are used to predict the future performance of the device. In this regard, it is possible that anesthesia agents could influence defibrillation energy requirements. Because of that possibility, a consistent anesthetic approach is clearly preferable. It has been shown in animal experiments that antiarrhythmic agents can affect defibrillation energy requirements [9]. Intraoperative use of antiarrhythmic agents is therefore not recommended unless required for patient stability. Therefore, avoidance of lidocaine, even as a local anesthetic agent, is advised. Also, general anesthetic agents may affect the induction of ventricular tachyarrhythmias [10–12].

After the surgeon has installed the lead system of the ICD, intraoperative testing of device function is performed in concert with the cardiac electrophysiologist. The sensing system is assessed for satisfactory signals that will allow adequate arrhythmia detection. Subsequently energy requirements for defibrillation (typically with brief cardiac application of alternating current) and an external cardioverter-defibrillator (ECD — CPI, St. Paul, MN) is utilized to deliver shocks to determine the minimum energy required for defibrillation. If 20 J or less reliably defibrillates, the pulse generator is then implanted. If energy requirements are higher, alternate patch positions or shocking lead polarity should be assessed to attempt to achieve lower defibrillation energy requirements. If attempts using the ECD fail, external "rescue" countershocks will be necessary and should always be anticipated. Depending upon the surgical approach, internal or external paddles may be necessary. Both should always be available and ready.

After the pulse generator is connected to the lead system, it is activated and appropriately programmed by the external programmer (with the wand placed through a sterile sleeve and positioned on the pulse generator). The device is then tested by again inducing ventricular fibrillation to ensure that both detection and therapy are satisfactory. After successful testing of the ICD pulse generator, the incisions are closed and the operative procedure is concluded. It is important to note that electrocautery can be sensed as ventricular fibrillation and result in inappropriate shocks [13]. Therefore after the generator is tested successfully, it should be deactivated prior to surgical closure if electrocautery is to be utilized.

Occasionally patient hemodynamic instability may limit fibrillation — defibrillation trials and it is important to carefully monitor patient status during the testing.

## Anesthesia for Patients with a Previously Implanted ICD

Anesthetic agents and techniques are again determined by the patient's condition and the planned operation. Electrocardiographic monitoring is imperative for all patients with an ICD undergoing surgery. As noted above, if electrocautery will be used, the ICD pulse generator should be incactivated with the programmer. If electrocautery is not planned and the ICD device remains active, an appropriate (toroid) magnet should be available for use should shock diversion become necessary. Any sustained ventricular arrhythmias occurring after device inactivation will require external cardiover-

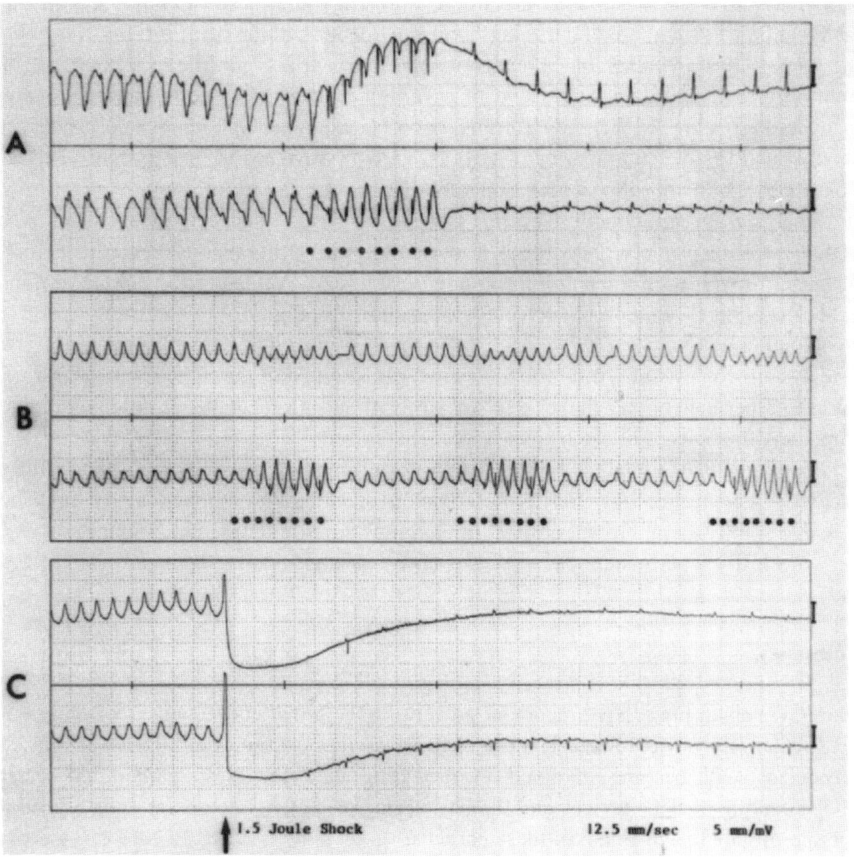


**Fig. 4 A–C.** Examples of tachycardia therapy from a multiprogrammable second generation ICD (Cadence, Ventritex Inc., Sunnyvale, California). In each panel two channel ambulatory ECG recordings are shown. In panel *A*, ventricular tachycardia is present in the left half of the tracing. It is successfully terminated by a burst of antitachycardia pacing stimuli. Panels *B* and *C* are continuous. In *B*, three attempts at antitachycardia pacing (eight stimuli each) are unsuccessful and ventricular tachycardia continues into panel *C* until a low energy cardioversion shock of 1.5 J (*arrow*) successfully restores sinus rhythm. Paper calibrations are 12.5 mm/s and 5 mm/mV, as shown

sion, which, therefore, should be immediately available. The presence of epicardial patch electrodes could result in some shielding of the heart from external defibrillation (the insulation on the back of the patches will block current flow). Therefore the current pathway for external defibrillation should be perpendicular to the implanted two patch electrodes in an anteroposterior orientation, and the sternal-apex external defibrillation approach is used [13].

## Future Developments

The currently approved ICD has undergone considerable evolutionary changes and will continue to be refined. Additionally, evolutionary approaches to implantation and tachycardia treatment are undergoing clinical evaluation at the present time. Currently the two major interests of investigational device trials are the development of multiprogrammable devices capable of a variety of tachyarrhythmic therapies (antitachycardia pacing, low energy cardioversion shocks, and high energy defibrillation shocks) and the development of nonthoracotomy approaches to lead system installation to obviate the need for a major operative procedure.

The multiprogrammable second generation devices appear most useful for patients whose primary arrhythmia is monomorphic ventricular tachycardia, which has been proven during electrophysiologic testing and evaluation to be pace terminable. The clinical function of such a device is shown in Fig. 4.

Nonthoracotomy lead system are also undergoing clinical evaluation [14]. The lead system consists of a transvenous catheter positioned in the right ventricular apex (akin to a permanent pacemaker ventricular lead) and a subcutaneous patch electrode (replacing the epicardial patch electrode).

With advances in delivered fibrillation waveforms [15], as well as further refinements in lead technology and miniaturization of electronic components, it may be possible some day to implant an ICD in the prepectoral region without major surgery, very much like a permanent pacemaker is now implanted.

## Summary

The ICD has an impressive record in preventing the lethal consequences of recurrent ventricular tachyarrhythmias. The use of these devices continues to increase and more physicians will become involved in providing care for these patients. A clear understanding of ICD devices and the basic principles of device operation is essential for appropriate management of these patients.

## References

1 Cobb LA, Werner JA, Trobaugh GB (1980) Sudden cardiac death II: Outcome of resuscitation, management and future connections. Mod Concepts Cardiovasc Dis 49:37–42

2 Mirowski M, Reid PR, Mower MM et al. (1980) Termination of malignant ventricular arrhythmias with an implanted defibrillator in human beings. N Engl J Med 303:322–324

3 Physician's manual (1989) Ventak™ P AICD™ model 1600 automatic implantable cardioverter-defibrillator, Cardiac Pacemakers, Inc., St. Paul MN, USA
4 Troup PJ, Chapman PD, Olinger GN, Kleinman LH (1985) The implanted defibrillator: Relation of defibrillating lead configuration and clinical variables to defibrillation threshold. J Am Coll Cardiol 6:1315–1321
5 Chapman PD (1986) Patient selection and preoperative evaluation for the implanted defibrillator. Clin Prog Electrophysiol Pacing 4:306–309
6 Winkle RA, Mead RH, Ruder MA et al. (1989) Long-term outcome with the automatic implantable cardioverter defibrillator. J Am Coll Cardiol 13:1353–1361
7 Tordjman-Fuchs T, Garan H, McGovern B et al. (1989) Out-of-hospital cardiac arrest: Improved long-term outcome in patients with automatic implantable cardioverter defibrillator (AICD). Circulation 80 [suppl II]:121 (abstract)
8 Lehmann MH, Steinman RT, Schuger CD, Jackson K (1988) The automatic implantable cardioverter defibrillator as antiarrhythmic treatment modality of choice for survivors of cardiac arrest unrelated to acute myocardial infarction. Am J Cardiol 62:803–805
9 Echt DS, Blach JN, Barbey JT, Coxe DR, Cato E (1989) Evaluation of antiarrhythmic drugs on defibrillation energy requirement in dogs. Sodium channel block and active potential prolongation. Circulation 75(5):1106–1117
10 Hunt GB, Ross DL (1988) Comparison of the effects of three anesthetic agents on induction of ventricular tachycardia in a canine model of myocardial infarction. Circulation 78:221–226
11 Denniss AR, Richards DA, Taylor AT, Uther JB (1989) Halothane anesthesia reduces inducibility of ventricular tachyarrhythmias in chronic canine myocardial infarction. Basic Res Cardiol 84:5–12
12 Deutsch N, Hantler CB, Tait AR, Uprichard A, Schork MA, Knight PR (1990) Suppression of ventricular arrhythmias by volatile anesthetics in a canine model of chronic myocardial infarction. Anesthesiology 72:1012–1021
13 Chapman PD, Veseth-Rogers JL, Duquette SE (1989) The implantable defibrillator and the emergency physician. Ann Emerg Med 18:579–585
14 Bach SM, Barstad J, Harper N et al. (1989) Initial clinical experience: ENDOTAK™ implantable transvenous defibrillator system. J Am Coll Cardiol 13:65A (abstract)
15 Chapman PD, Souza JJ, Wetherbee JN, Troup PJ (1989) Comparison of monophasic and single and dual capacitor biphasic waveforms for nonthoracotomy canine internal defibrillation. J Am Coll Cardiol 14:242–245

# Electromagnetic Interference and Cardiac Pacemakers

I.M.G. Bourgeois

## Introduction

Pacemaker malfunction due to adverse effects of external factors on pacemaker function were first observed during the early phase of clinical pacemaker use. Lillihey, who used external (mains-powered) pacemakers for the postoperative management of children who had undergone cardiac surgery in the 1950s, lost patients due to mains failures in the Minnesota power plants. As a result, he asked his engineer, Earl Bakken, to design the first battery-powered cardiac pacemaker. This was the initial technical step towards making the function of pacemakers less dependent on external influences.

Early models of implantable demand pacemakers raised additonal questions additional how to make pacemakers safe and reliable in the presence of interference. This need became even more important with the development of atrial-triggered, ventricular demand pacemakers [1]. Such pacemakers should be designed so that interference detected by the atrial amplifier does not trigger stimulation of the ventricle at an inappropriate moment during the cardiac cycle. Similarly, with unipolar implantable antitachycardia devices, electrical stimulation therapy should not be delivered in the presence of interference [2].

Now more than 250,000 pacemakers are implanted yearly worldwide. Pacemaker patients travel throughout the world and are exposed to different electromagnetic fields in their daily life as well as in the hospital where they may be receiving therapy for some other condition [3]. How a pacemaker detects and reacts to different types of electromagnetic interference (EMI) and identification of potential EMI sources that could affect pacemaker behaviour are important concerns for clinicians.

## The Pacemaker Detection System

A demand pacemaker system has a detection circuit to sense the intrinsic heart activity. The intrinsic heart activity occurs as the myocardial cells depolarize. The myocardium has a special structure in which one cell depolarizes, triggering the depolarization of adjacent cells. The resulting depolarization wave (electrogram) leads to the mechanical contraction of the heart. The depolarization wavefront, which passes under the electrode in contact with myocardium, is sensed by the pulse generator, via the lead. The depolarization wave, or electrogram is detected by the electrode as a slow, varying voltage when the wavefront is still distant. When the depolarization dipole passes under the electrode there is a rapid, varying electrical signal (the intrinsic deflection). As the wavefront goes away this signal decays to the baseline (figure 1). The electrogram can be characterized by its amplitude (maximum peak-to-peak voltage difference in the electrogram), its slew rate, (maximum voltage change per second) and its frequency content (spectral distribution of frequencies in the electrogram). The frequency distribution peaks around 20 to 30 Hz (Fig. 2) [6].

These characteristics define the design of the sensing amplifier of the pulse generator. The QRS electrogram is amplified via a bandpass filter, centered around 30 Hz. The amplified signal is transmitted to a detection circuit, which reacts to a minimum amplitude level (0.5 to 20 mV) and a minimum slew rate (0.1 to 4.0 V/s)

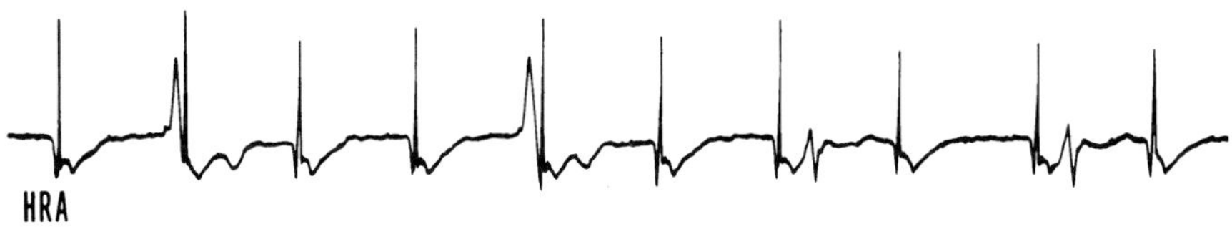


**Fig. 1.** High right atrial electrogram (*HRA*) with the *narrow lines* corresponding to the intrinsic deflection. The far-field QRS complex is seen just prior to the second and the fifth, and just following the seventh and ninth intrinsic deflections. (From [31] with permission of Futura Publishing Company)

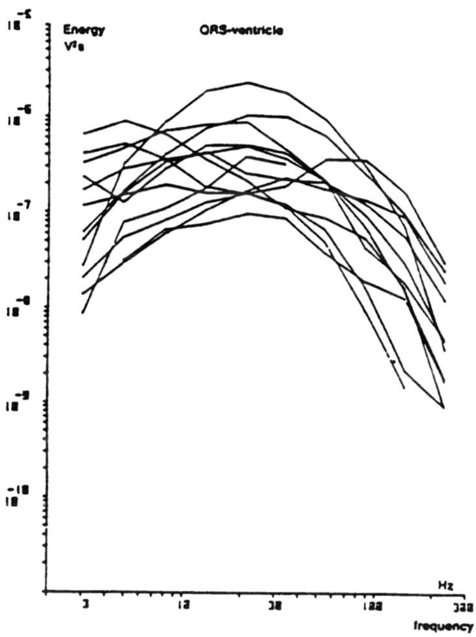


**Fig. 2** The frequency power spectrum of the QRS electrogram. The maximum peak is around 30 Hz. (From [6], with permission of Futura Publishing Company)

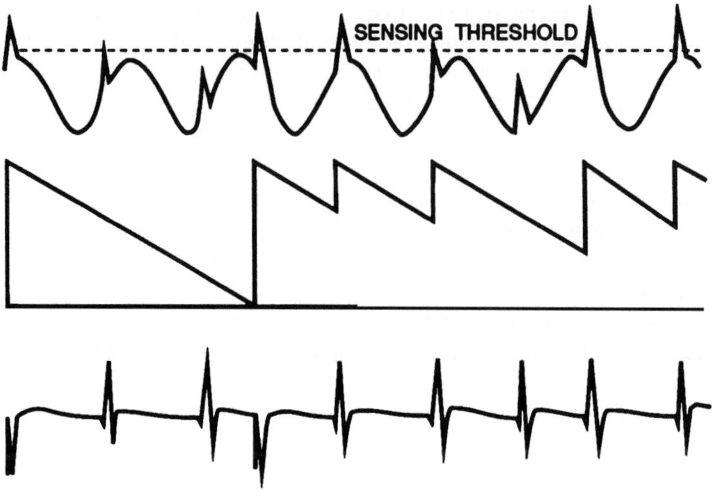


**Fig. 3.** The *upper panel* depicts the sensed electrogram superimposed on a background of continuous interference, the *middle panel* the signal from the timer of the pacemaker circuit, and the *lower panel* a simulated electrocardiographic signal. The first complex is a paced ventricular complex. The two following complexes have not been detected by the amplifier since, due to continuous interference, they did not reach the sensing threshold. The fourth complex is a paced ventricular complex. The fifth and sixth complexes are sensed, since they exceed the sensing threshold and reset the timing circuit. (From [31] with permission of Futura Publishing Company)

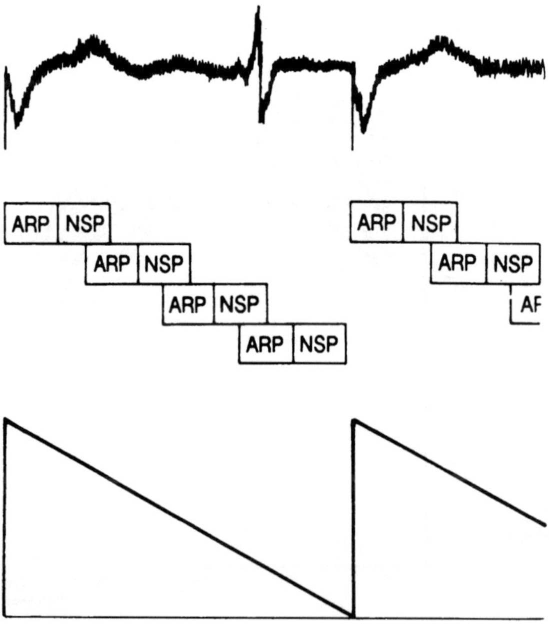


**Fig. 4.** Surface EGC, tracing with a sequence of absolute refractory periods (*ARP*) and noise-sensing periods (*NSP*) provided by a pacemaker. The *lower panel* shows the timing circuit of the pacemaker. The first complex is a paced ventricular complex. In the middle of the first noise sampling period, the amplifier senses a signal which resets ARP, but not the timing circuit. During the following two NSP, extraneous signals are again detected. Following the fourth NSP, the pacemaker escapes. This demonstrates a mechanism by which the pacemaker can switch to an asynchronous mode in the presence of continuous interference. (From [31] with permission of Futura Publishing Company)

[7]. Pacemakers of some manufacturers store the amplitude of continous interference in their detection circuit and detect the rapid electrogram amplitude change versus the stored interference level (Fig. 3).

Pulse generators are designed so that they cannot sense any signals following a cardiac event, during which time the cardiac cells are depolarized and sensing of a cardiac event is physiologically impossible. Such a period, termed the absolute refractory or blanking period, starts with each cardiac event and has a duration of 100 to 150 ms. The absolute refractory period avoids sensing of extraneous signals during a specified part of the cardiac cycle. Another protection mechanism built into the pulse generator by manufacturers is the relative refractory or noise sampling period, which starts at the end of the absolute refractory period. This prevents an inappropriately long asystole caused by interference from unwanted, extraneous signals. Sensed events during this relative refractory period do not reset the lower rate counter, but will restart a new absolute refractory period. During the relative refractory period, it is highly unlikely for a sensed event to be due to sensed intrinsic heart activity. More likely, the sensed event is due to other factors, such as signals from interference or due to repolarization (T-wave sensing). Continous interference will lead to asynchronous pacing (Fig. 4). The duration of the noise sampling period is roughly 130 ms, which permits low frequency rejection down to 8 Hz. This frequency is generated by electrodiesel converters in railroad engines. Pulsed interference may or may not result in prolongation of the basic pacing rate (Fig. 5).

A sensing amplifier has its limitations. It is especially affected by high input of signals which can saturate it. The level of input influences the sensing characteristics

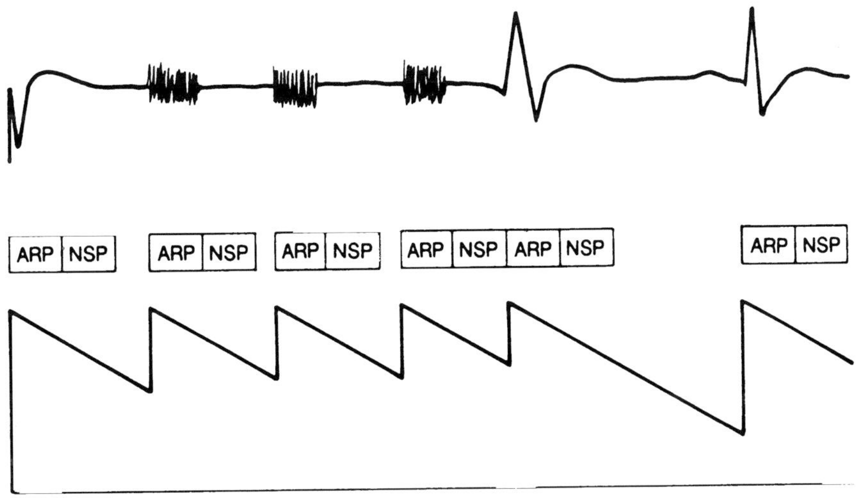


**Fig. 5** The *upper panel* shows a simulated ECG with three bursts of pulsed interference, the *middle panel* absolute refractory (*ARP*) and noise-sensing periods (*NSP*) and the *lower panel* the pacemaker timing circuit. The three pulsed interferences, as well as the two last QRS complexes, are sensed outside the ARP and NSP, resulting in the resetting of the timing circuit. These three interference signals have caused a period of asystole. (From [31] with permission of Futura Publishing Company)

of a pulse generator. At low interference levels, when the spontaneous electrogram is greater than the interference level, every depolarization is detected. If the amplifier is saturated by extraneous signals, however, the detection circuit will not reset the lower rate counter and the pacemaker system will function in the asynchronous mode. For interference levels between those extremes, the detection of spontaneous events depends on the phase angle of the interference signal and the electrogram (Fig. 3). Thus, there can be partial reversion to the asynchronous mode of pacing. Figure 6 depicts these various types of sensing behaviour.

The electrical signal detected by the sensing amplifier should be only the QRS complex of the electrocardiogram. The sensitivity of the pulse generator to interference by EMI or skeletal muscle myopotentials can be significantly reduced by using a bipolar rather than a unipolar electrode [8]. Pacemakers with bipolar leads are relatively insensitive to EMI [9]. The induced voltage at the sensing amplifier is directly proportional to the surface area of the pathway of the induced current (Lenz's law). This current pathway is from the amplifier terminal to the electrode coil, through the electrode tip to the blood and/or tissue, and then to the indifferent electrode. With

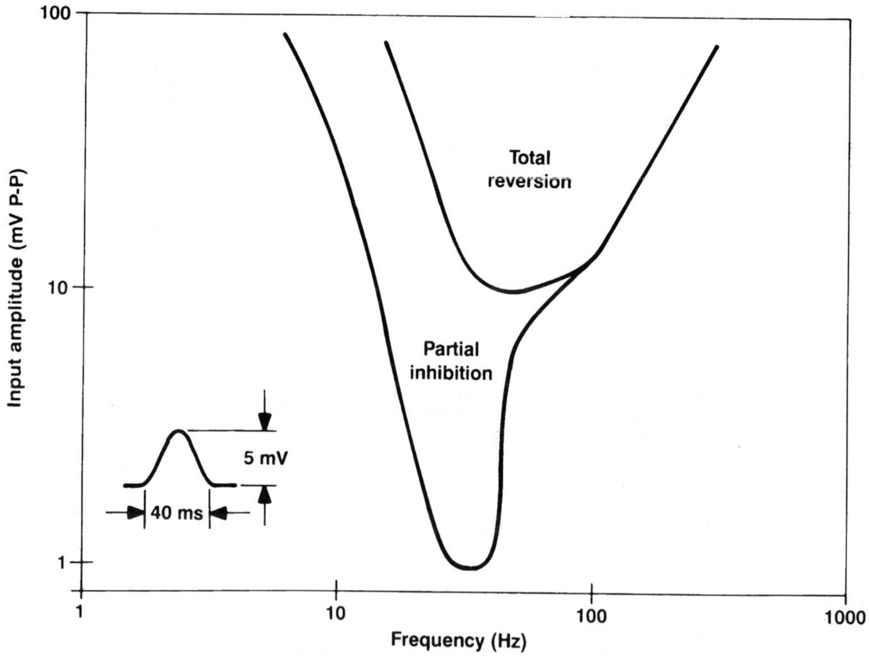


**Fig. 6.** The frequency of continuous interference is depicted along the horizontal axis, the peak-to-peak amplitude of continuous interference along the vertical axis. A sine square test signal, simulating an electrogram, has been superimposed on the continuous interference. The amplifier senses every test signal in all areas below the curves. In the area marked *partial inhibition*, the circuit senses some test signals. In the area marked *total reversion*, the amplifier senses no signals

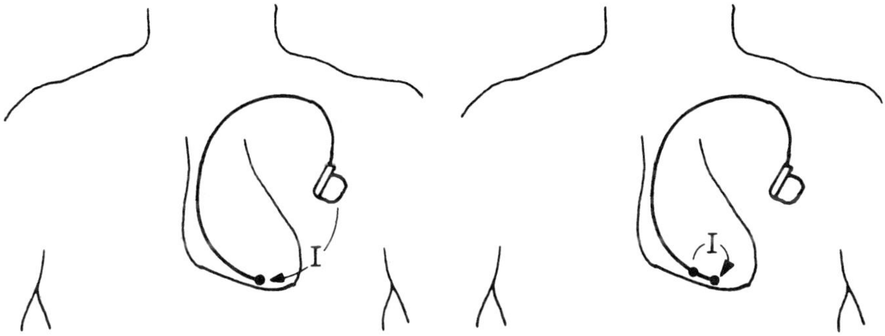


**Fig. 7.** The *left side* of the figure depicts a unipolar pacemaker lead system with a pulse generator implanted in the pectoral area. The current flows from the pacemaker can through the tissue to the electrode tip and back via the electrode to the pulse generator. The *circle* delineates the area in which electromagnetic interference (*I*) can be sensed. On the *right side*, a bipolar pacemaker lead system is shown. Current flows only between the two electrodes, so that the surface area of the circle is much smaller than for a unipolar system. (From [31] with permission of Futura Publishing Company).

bipolar leads, this area is rather small since the electrode tip and indifferent electrode are close together. In contrast, with unipolar leads the pulse generator acts as the indifferent electrode and is quite remote from the electrode tip (Fig. 7).

## Factors Affecting Pacemaker Behavior

The most common factors which influence pulse generator behavior are electromagnetic fields and myopotentials. Mechanical forces, electrostatic discharges, radiation and some patient medications can also affect pacemaker function.

### *Mechanical Influences on Pacemaker Function*

It is well known that lead dislodgement, requiring prompt intervention, can occur in the immediate postoperative period following pacemaker implantation. Such early dislodgement can be caused by arm and thorax movement during the recovery phase. Careful testing of sensing and pacing thresholds during implantation should reduce the risk of dislodgement, as should the use of tined or screw-in myocardial electrodes.

Pulse generators can withstand subatmospheric pressures. Testing with high vacuum levels is standard procedure during the production cycle. The pacemaker can could be deformed if it is subjected to pressures around 1 kg/cm$^2$, as would occur when diving at 10 m below water level. Pacemaker can deformation could result in pacemaker dysfunction, and pacemaker patients should be advised to abstain from deep-water diving.

Pacemakers are designed to withstand vibration forces up to at least three times that of the force of the earth's gravity. Only astronauts and test pilots are exposed to higher accelerations. Pacemakers are also capable of resisting a shock equivalent to several hundred times that of the earth's gravity.

A car seat belt will not affect the pulse generator, but can create some discomfort by pressing on the pulse generator pocket. Nevertheless, following a serious car accident, the pacemaker system and area surrounding the pulse generator should be checked by a physician.

Ultrasound imaging waves have a low energy that should not affect pacemakers. Lithotripsy shocks, however, should be delivered in synchrony with the QRS, as these shock waves could stimulate the heart. In vitro tests have shown pacemaker inhibiton, with no damage to the pulse generator in the models of one manufacturer, while some reports indicate inhibition, reprogramming, or even output failure. Pacemaker patients should be carefully monitored during lithotripsy [10–12].

Placing an electronic vibrator over pulse generators, in which the stimulation rate control algorithm employs a piezo crystal sensor, could result in a high stimulation rate. With such devices, vibrations received while driving a car induce only a small increase in stimulation rate. Further, the energy content of pulsed ultrasound waves used for imaging purposes is too low to alter paced rates. Lithrotripsy shock waves, however, could increase paced rates with such pacing systems (Irnich et al., this volume).

Rate-adaptive pacemakers, in which the stimulation rate is controlled by variations in intrathoracic impedance could increase their stimulation rate as a result of rapid thoracic movements, as with tachyapnea or mechanical ventilators or arm movements.

## Interference Which Could Affect Pacemaker Function in Daily Life

### *Electromagnetic Fields*

Electromagnetic fields created by mains power sources should not affect bipolar pacing systems. With unipolar systems, small voltages induced by these electromagnetic fields (50 Hz in Europe, 60 Hz in the USA) is partially filtered out by the bandpass amplifier (Fig. 6). Continuous low level interference from mains power has little effect on pacemakers, but strong fields will cause the pacemaker to revert to asynchronous pacing (interference mode).

Electromagnetic fields created by household appliances, such as electric razors, hair dryers, vacuum cleaners, washing machines, microwaves, radio, television, electric blankets and heating pads should not affect pacemaker function. However, moving a razor or a vibrator over the pulse generator implantation site could lead to pacemaker inhibition. Such movement would generate a varying electromagnetic field, which might affect the pacemaker in a similar manner to low frequency, pulsed electromagnetic fields.

Interference from high frequency fields, such as microwave ovens and radio frequency remote control devices for garage door openers and burglar alarms, are generally safe. Home radio transmission devices are safe if they conform to national standards for such devices.

Pulsed electromagnetic interference, with repetition frequencies of between 1 and roughly 5 Hz, inhibits pacemakers. This can occur when the patient is standing close to a rotating radar or passing through some models of older metal detector gates [13]. Such incidental inhibition of demand pacemaker function should be rather benign, provided asystole does not last longer then 3–5 s.

Detection of pulsed interference by pacemakers whose ventricular output is triggered by sensed events could induce arrhythmias in patients with ischemic heart disease or acute acid-base or electrolyte imbalance. Ventricular triggered pacemakers should therefore be programmed with a long refractory period (i.e., 400 ms) to avoid stimulation during the vulnerable phase. The use of bipolar leads with a triggered pacing system is strongly recommended to minimize interference detection.

With atrial-synchronized ventricular pacing (VDD), pulsed interference could be sensed by the more sensitive atrial amplifiers, resulting in ventricular pacing and arrhythmias [14]. Induced arrhythmias can be minimized by using bipolar leads and by programming the ventricular upper rate to 150 bpm or lower. Alternatively, the atrial refractory period can be programmed to 400 ms or longer.

Pulsed interference in a VDD pacing system can also induce a pacemaker-mediated tachycardia, with a rate close to the upper rate of the pacing system [15]. In this case the atrial amplifier detects the interference and triggers a ventricular stimulus. The resulting ventricular depolarization could be conducted retrogradely to the atrium via the AV node or an accessory pathway [17]. Retrograde (VA) conduction times can vary from 150 to over 400 ms. If this atrial depolarization is detected by the atrial amplifier, it triggers a ventricular stimulus. If the latter process perpetuates itself, a tachycardia is produced (Fig. 8). Such pacemaker-mediated tachycardia can be avoided by programming a postventricular atrial refractory period longer than

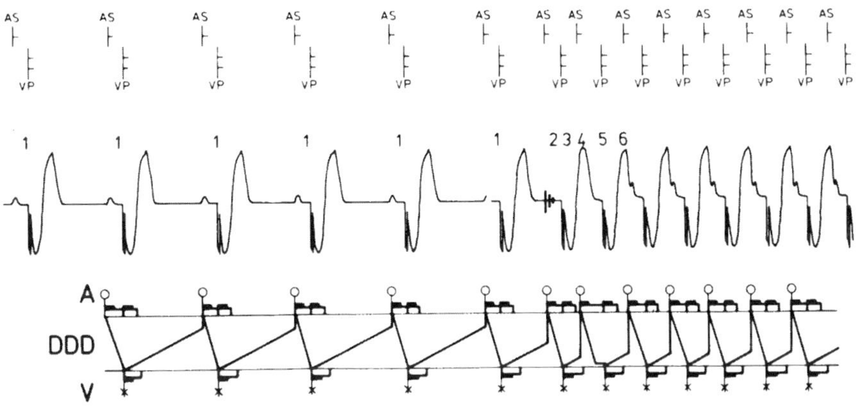


**Fig. 8.** Simulated ECG of a dual chamber (*DDD*) pacemaker. The *upper panel* shows the marker channel, the *middle panel* a simulated surface ECG, and the *lower panel* a ladder diagram (*AS*, atrial sensing; VP, ventricular pacing). P-waves (*1*) induce normal atrial-synchronous, ventricular triggered stimulation. Noise (*2*) is detected by the atrial sensing amplifier, resulting in ventricular stimulation (*3*). In the T-wave of that stimulated complex is a concealed, retrograde P-wave (*4*) which is sensed in the atrium. The AV delay is then prolonged because of the upper rate limit, resulting in a stimulated complex (*5*). Process repeats itself with the next sensed, nonconcealed, retrograde P-wave (*6*), thereby producing a pacemaker-mediated tachycardia

the retrograde (VA) conduction time. Some authors have reported cases in which the retrograde P-wave has a lower amplitude than a normal P-wave [15, 16]. In this case, reprogramming atrial sensitivity could be used to avoid detection of retrograde P-waves while still detecting normal sinus P-waves. Some dual-chamber pacing systems will automatically drop every seventh ventricular stimulus when operating at their upper rate limit. This could terminate pacemaker-mediated tachycardia.

With dual-chamber, rate-responsive pacemakers, the atrial rate can be validated by the sensor output. If there is significant discrepancy between the sensed atrial rate and the rate indicated by the sensor, the pacing system stops tracking the atrial signal, thus avoiding pacemaker-induced tachycardias.

Transcutaneous nerve stimulators, as used for pain control or for weight loss, could affect pacemakers by inhibiting or triggering output, or switching the device to asynchronous operation [17].

Industrial equipment with high power requirements could inhibit pacing systems or cause them to revert to asynchronous operation. On-site testing is recommended if pacemaker patients are likely to come in close proximity to induction furnaces, electrical welding equipment, power transformers or power lines. Programming unipolar, single-chamber pacemakers to the triggered mode should be considered if the patients regularly come in the vicinity of such installations. Dual-chamber systems should also be checked with care on site. It is strongly recommended that the patient be carefully interviewed prior to implantation to establish the likelihood of exposure to such strong fields. A bipolar lead system should be selected in the case of regular exposure.

### *Electrostatic Field*

Touch control systems have electrostatic fields which, when activated, create currents which could be sensed by a pacemaker as a single sensed event. This is a rather benign occurrence with ventricular demand pacemakers, but could be dangerous with triggered ventricular pacemakers if they are not programmed to a low maximum pacing rate, i.e., less than 150 bpm.

### *Myopotentials and T-wave Sensing*

With pectoral implants, depending on the implantation technique, skeletal myopotentials are present on the pacemaker can. With unipolar pacemaker systems, skeletal myopotentials contaminate the sensed electrocardiogram and can lead to mypotential inhibition. Myopotential inhibition with unipolar pacemaker system has been reported to vary between 20% and 80%. In most cases it is rather benign. Myopotential inhibition can be avoided by implanting a bipolar system, by implanting the generator in a Parsonnet pouch, or by positioning the uncoated area of the pacemaker can opposite to the muscle [9, 18].

T-wave sensing during the relative refractory period will not affect the pacemaker escape rate. Such sensing after the relative refractory period will result in a prolonged escape interval (pacing at a lower rate then programmed).

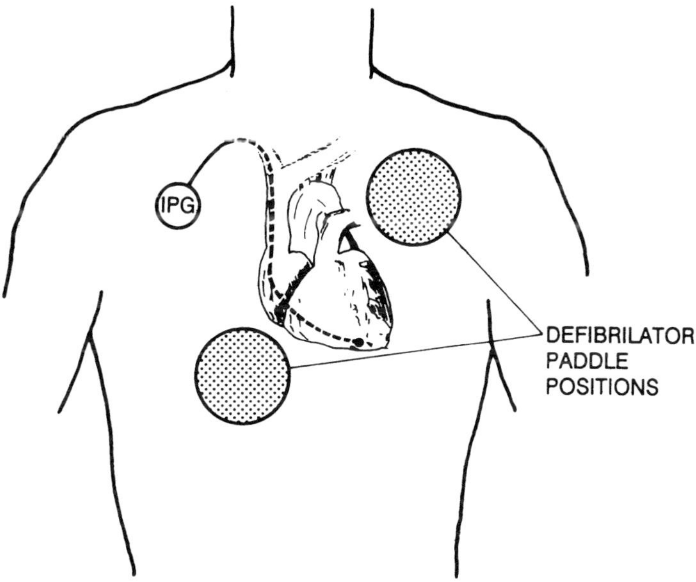


**Fig. 9.** Preferred defibrillator paddle positions for transthoracic defibrillation or cardioversion. One should avoid placing the defibrillator paddle over the pulse generator or along the line of axis of the pulse generator and pacing electrode. (From [31] with permission of Futura Publishing Company)

## Interference in the Hospital Environment

### *Defibrillation*

The extremely high transthoracic currents used with external cardioversion or defibrillation could damage the pacing system [19]. The current could induce an electromagnetic field which, in a unipolar system, could produce a high current through the electrode. This could damage the tissue under the electrode tip, resulting in temporary or permanent malsensing. While the induced current is shorted over a protection circuit within the pulse generator, it still could create a significant voltage there which could reprogram or damage the pulse generator. Consequently, pacemaker systems should be checked by a physician after any defibrillation or cardioversion. The induced current can be minimized by placing the defibrillation paddles perpendicular to the axis of the pulse generator and the pacing electrode (Fig. 9).

### *Diathermy, Electrocautery, and Electrocoagulation*

If not detected during the noise sampling window, these modulated high frequency fields could be detected by demand pacemakers causing them to revert to asynchronous operation. Alternatively they could trigger rapid paced rates with triggered pacemakers. Diathermy or electrocautery/electrocoagulation could also damage the insulation of the electrode leading to malsensing or ineffective stimulation and should not be performed in close proximity to the pulse generator itself. Bipolar diathermy and electrocautery/electrocoagulation are preferred, and monitoring of the patient's pulse or heart sounds is recommended during such interventions [20].

### *Nuclear Magnetic Resonance*

These strong magnetic fields could switch the pulse generator to the asynchronous mode of operation. There are reports that triggered pacemakers track pulsed radiofrequency fields. The response to nuclear magnetic resonance fields will likely vary among different pacemaker models. Nevertheless, overall pacemaker reliability seems not to be affected by nuclear magnetic resonance imaging equipment [21, 22].

### *Pacemakers Programmers and Other Stimulators*

Modern pacemaker programmers emit searching signals for the establishement of the bidirectional telemetry link. Before the reed switch closes, such search signals could be detected by sensing electrodes, possibly resulting in pacemaker inhibition with a demand system or initiation of tachycardia with a triggered system. Implantable neuromuscular pulse generators emit a burst of stimuli which could be sensed by the amplifier. The implantation of a bipolar pacing system is recommended for patients with implantable neuromuscular or transcutaneous nerve stimulators [23].

### *Ionizing Radiation*

The semiconductor circuits of the pulse generator appear quite sensitive to ionizing beams of radiation. Of these circuits, the digital control circuit is most sensitive. The effect of similar radiation doses on different models of pulse generator models varies widely: some are hardly affected, others show a shift in programmed parameters, and others fail catastrophically. Diagnostic radiation (X-ray) doses are so low that they should not be of any concern. With therapeutic radiation doses, however, the pacemaker should be shielded and carefully assessed at intervals during and after completion of the course of radiation therapy [24].

### *Medication*

Pacing thresholds are influenced by drugs, electrolyte balance and the neuroendocrine system [25–29]. Steroids and cathecolamines lower pacing thresholds, whereas β-adrenergic blockers and some antiarrhythmic agents (e.g., flecanaide) increase pacing thresholds. Volatile anesthetic agents, such as halothane, may affect pacing thresholds [30].

## Conclusions

Understanding the behavior of pacemakers in the presence of interference is complex and requires substantial knowledge of the pacing system and its programmed settings.

Potential sources of interference may be difficult to identify and quantify. Interference signals may combine with myopotentials, producing an augmented signal which inhibits or triggers pulse generator output. Modern pacing systems, fortunately, are relatively insensitive to mechanical or electromagnetic interference. Consequently, inhibition or altered pacing during exposure to most types of interference is self-limited and effects of any malfunction relatively benign. Bipolar pacing systems appear much more immune to external interference and should be preferred to unipolar systems, particularly with expected repeated exposure to noisy environments.

## References


1 Bourgeois IM (1981) Some engineering aspects of physiological pacing. In: Obel IWP (ed) Physiological pacing. Pittman Medical, Bath, pp 84–100

2 Calkins H, Brinker J, Veltri EP, Guarneri T, Levine JH (1990) Clinical interactions between pacemakers and automatic implantable cardioverter-defibrillator. J Am Coll Cardiol 16:666–673

3 Hardage ML, Marbach JR, Winsor DW (1985) The pacemaker patient in the therapeutic and diagnostic device environment. In: Barold S (ed) Modern cardiac pacing. Futura, New York, pp 857–873

4 Myers GH, Kresh YM, Parsonnet V (1978) Characteristics of intracardiac electrograms. PACE 1:90–103

5 Parsonnet V, Myers GH, Kresh YM (1980) Characteristics of intracardiac electrograms II: atrial endocardial electrogram. PACE 3:406–417

6 Kleinert M, Elmquist H, Strandberg H (1979) Spectral properties of atrial and ventricular endocardial signals. PACE 2:11–19

7 Ohm OJ (1979) The interdependence between electrogram, total electrode impedance and pacemaker input impedance necessary to obtain adequate functioning of demand pacemakers. PACE 2:465–485

8 DeCaprio V, Hurzeler P, Furman S (1977) A comparison of unipolar and bipolar electrograms for cardiac pacemaker sensing. Circulation 56:750–755

9 Fetter J, Bobeldyk GL, Engman FJ (1984) The clinical incidence and significance of myopotential sensing with unipolar pacemakers. PACE 7:871–881

10 Cooper D, Wilkoff B, Masterson M, Castle L, Belko K, Simmons T, Morant V, Streen S, Maloney J (1988) Effects of extracorporeal shock wave lithotripsy on cardiac pacemakers and its safety in patients with implanted cardiac pacemakers. PACE 11:1607–1616

11 Fetter J, Patterson D, Aram G, Hayes DL (1989) Effects of extracorporeal shock wave lithotripsy on single chamber rate response and dual chamber pacemakers. PACE 12:1494–1501

12 Ector H, Janssen L, Baert L, De Geest (1989) Extracorporeal shock wave lithotripsy and cardiac arrhythmias. PACE 12:1910–1917

13 Cooperman Y, Zarfati D, Laniado S (1988) The effect of metal detector gates on implanted permanent pacemakers. PACE 11:1386–1387

14 Fröhlig G, Schwerdt H, Schieffer H, Bette L (1988) Atrial signal variations and pacemaker malsensing during exercise: a study in the time and frequency domain. J Am Coll Cardiol 11:806–813

15 Den Dulk K, Lindemans FW, Bär FW, Wellens HJJ (1982) Pacemaker related tachycardias. PACE 5:476–485

16 Den Dulk K, Lindemans FW, Wellens HJJ (1984) Management of pacemaker circus movement tachycardias. PACE 7:346–355

17 Rasmussen MJ, Hayes DL, Vlietstra RE, Thorsteinson G (1988) Can transcutaneous electrical nerve stimulation be safely used in patients with permanent cardiac pacemakers? Mayo Clin Proc 63:443–445

pacemakers assessed by ambulatory holter monitoring of the electrocardiogram. PACE 3:470–478
19 Levine PA (1985) Effect of cardioversion and defibrillation on implanted cardiac pacemakers. In: Barold S (ed) Modern cardiac pacing. Futura, New York, pp 875–886
20 Levine PA, Baladfy GJ, Lazar HJ, Belott PH, Roberts AJ (1986) Electrocautery and pacemakers: management of the paced patient subject ot electrocautery. Am Thorac Surg 41:313–317
21 Erlebacher JA, Cahill PT, Pannizzo F, Knowles RJ (1986) Effect of magnetic resonance imaging on DDD pacemakers. Am J Cardiol 57:437–440
22 Fetter J, Aram G, Holmes DR, Gray JE, Hayes DL (1984) The effects of nuclear magnetic resonance imagers on external and implantable pulse generators. PACE 7:720–727
23 Anderson C, Oxhoj H, Arnbo P (1990) Management of spinal cord stimulators in patients with cardiac pacemakers. PACE 13:574–577
24 Salmi J, Eskola HJ, Pitkaenen MA, Malmivuo JAV (1990) The influence of electromagnetic interference and ionizing radiation on cardiac pacemakers. Strahlenther Onkol 166:153–155
25 Dohrman ML, Goldschlager N (1985) Metabolic and pharmacologic effects on myocardial stimulation thresholds in patients with cardiac pacemakers. In: Barold S (ed) Modern cardiac pacing. Futura, New York, pp 161–170
26 Falk RH, Knowlton AA, Battinelli NJ (1988) The effect of propanolol and verapamil on external pacing threshold: a placebo-controlled study. PACE 11:1439–1443
27 Preston TA, Fletcher RD, Lucchesi BR, Judge RD (1967) Changes in myocardial threshold. Physiological and pharmacologic factors in patients with implanted pacemakers. Am Heart J 74:235–242
28 Saoudi N, Berland J, Hocq R, Cave D, Cribrier A, Letac B (1987) Comparison des effets de l'ajmaline et de la procainamide dans le diagnostic du block auricolo-ventriculaire proxystique. Ann Cardiol Angeiol (Paris) 36:13–17
29 Siddons H, Sowton E (1967) Effect of drugs on stimulation thresholds. In: Siddons H, Sowton E (eds) Cardiac pacemakers. Thomas, Springfield, pp 168–169
30 Zaidan JR, Curling PE, Craver JM (1985) Effect of enflurane, isoflurane and halothane on pacing stimulation thresholds in men. PACE 8:32–34
31 Sutton R, Bourgeois IM (1991) Foundations of cardiac pacing: an illustrated practical guide in basic pacing, vol 1. Futura, New York

# Radiofrequency Transmission and Cardiac Pacemakers

T. BOSSERT

## Introduction

Telegraph and radiofrequency (longwave, medium wave, shortwave) broadcasting stations have been in operation for over half a century. Some of these facilities are assigned to transmit worldwide and must be operated with high transmitted power (field strenghts), sometimes exceeding 1 MW. As the field strenght may be very high in the immediate surroundings of radiofrequency broadcasting stations, limits for the allowable exposure to radiofrequency fields were established early. For example, allowable exposure limits in Germany are set forth in DIN/VDE 0848 by the national standard committee "Deutsches Institut für Normung", and in the United States in ANSI C95.1 provided by the American National Standards Institute. Concerning exposure limits, broadcasting companies must provide fences around transmitting facilities. Depending on power and frequency of transmission, fences may surround areas from 400 $m^2$ to more than 100,000 $m^2$.

If a pacemaker is constructed so that it is compatible with allowable exposure limits, permanent radiofrequency transmitters should not pose a problem for pacemaker patients. On the other hand, miniaturization of electronic circuits has enabled the use of mobile transmitters. These could be hazardous to pacemaker patients. Further, since mobile transmitters may be carried directly on the body, transmission power output from these sources must be restricted to only a few watts for pacemaker patients.

## Biohazards

Recommended limits for radiofrequency broadcast transmission (e.g., DIN/VDE 0848 and ANSI C95.1) were intended for healthy people without implanted pacemakers. With high frequency transmission, exceeded limits may cause whole-body hyperthermia. At frequencies below longwave, tissue irritation effects predominate. It is more difficult to estimate biohazards to pacemaker patients caused by radiofrequency or electromagnetic fields, since other factors come into play.

On the one hand, the implanted pacemaker lead is a conducter in direct contact with the heart. With higher frequency radiotransmission, whole-body hyperthermia may be less a problem than burns to the myocardium. With lower frequencies, myocardial irritation effects might be the cause for ventricular arrhythmias or fibrillation. On the other hand, the pacemaker circuitry might be susceptible to radiofrequency or electromagnetic interference; in which case, the implanted lead would act as an antenna and supply the pulse generator with a high frequency interference voltage. This could lead to pacemaker inhibition and perhaps even destroy or damage some of its more sensitive components.

## Radiofrequency Transmission on Pacemaker Patients

At the Institut für Rundfunktechnik, experiments have been carried out to determine the effects of radiofrequency transmission in pacemaker patients. The first step was to find out how the pacemaker lead functions as an antenna in a dummy body. The human trunk was simulated by a tank 52 cm high with an oval cross-section of 34 x 18 cm. The tank was filled with NaCl solution of 0.5 S/m conductivity. Results suggested a resonance at 10–50 MHZ and a high antenna gain for magnetic fields, but a good shielding against high frequency electric fields provided by dissipative body tissue.

The second step was to test 40 different types of cardiac pacemakers for their interference pattern. Results agreed with unpublished testing of 119 pacemakers models by TÜV Essen [1]. The tolerated interference levels show a large variance. For example, at 1 MHZ some models of pacemakers are almost a 1000 times more sensitive to electromagnetic interference than others. Unfortunately, in all our tests not a single model of pacemaker met the requirements of DIN/VDE 0848 and ANSI C95.1 completely. Additionally, contrary to assertions by pacemaker manufacturers that devices would revert to asynchronous operation with strong radiofrequency transmission interference, all pacemakers could be inhibited temporarily by adequately modulated radio signals.

## Recommendations

Based on our findings, safe distances (estimated worst case situation) from a radiofrequency transmission source for patients with pacemakers compared to those without are provided in Table 1. This worst situation means simultaneously the worst orientation of the lead in the field, the worst modulation of the transmitter, and the worst pacemaker type with respect to the transmitted frequency in a patient who is pacemaker dependent. Since the probability of the latter combination is small, the information in Table 1 is probably more of theoretical interest. Nevertheless, it can be seen from Table 1 that shortwave transmitters should pose, if indeed at all, the greatest risk of complications. With mobile radio transmitters, distances are much shorter. However, these shorter distances cannot be neglected, because the pacemaker patient may not be aware of a mobile transmitting radiofrequency source close to him.

**Table 1.** Least distances (worst case situation) from radiofrequency transmitting sources to avoid problems with interference (patients with pacemaker) or hyperthermia/irritation (person without pacemaker)

| Radiofrequency | | Patient with pacemaker | Person without pacemaker |
|---|---|---|---|
| Powerful radio stations | LW | 600 m | << 5 m |
| | MW | 1 500 m | 10 m |
| | SW | 10 000 m | 200 m |
| Mobile radio sets | | 3 – 20 m | Body surface |

LW, longwave; MW, medium wave; SW, short wave

## Conclusions

National and international standards are currently being recommended and tested to make pacemakers fail-safe against all radiofrequency interferences. However, since no valid standards exist at present, the implanting physician should forewarn the patient of potential hazards from radiofrequency transmission sources. Moreover, it is the responsibility of pacemaker manufacturers to inform implanting physicians in some detail about the fail-safe features of specific devices. However, it may be inappropriate to make global statements, since various models of pacemakers may have different fail-saife features. Finally, if the pacemaker manufacturer cannot provide useful information concerning the safety of a particular device when exposed to radiofrequency transmission, the physicians is advised to assume the worst case situation (Table 1) for that manufacturer's model of pacemaker.

## References

1 Bossert T, Dahme M (1988) Hazards from electromagnetic fields; influence on cardiac pacemakers by powerful radio transmitters. Sixth International Conference on Electromagnetic Compatibility. Institution of Electronic and Radio Engineers, London (Publication no 81)

# Nuclear Magnetic Resonance Imaging in Pacemaker Patients

F. IBERER, E. JUSTICH, K.H. TSCHELIESSNIGG AND A. WASLER

## Introduction

The manufacturers of nuclear magnetic resonance (NMR) scanners [1], as well as the manufacturers of pacemakers, emphasize that NMR tomography of pacemaker patients is contraindicated. However, NMR results, required for planning oncologic and surgical procedures, cannot be obtained by other methods. Nevertheless, the possible risk of pacemaker malfunction due to NMR has to be taken into consideration.

A number of observations of possible interactions between NMR scanners and pacemakers have been published [2–6]. Chauvin and co-workers have observed pacemaker function (V00 and VVI modes) during NMR tomography [2]. Pulse amplitudes and frequencies of time-varying magnetic fields have been reported to resemble cardiac myopotentials [2, 6]. Furthermore, rapid cardiac stimulation [5] and malfunction [3] have also been described.

Following in vitro experiments using a variety of Medtronic and Biotronic pacemakers and pacemaker leads [7, 8], investigations of the effects of NMR in pacemaker patients were carried out by the Departments of Surgery and Radiology at the University of Graz, Austria [9, 10]. The models of pacemakers and lead systems tested are listed in Table 1. For all investigations the Phillips Gyroscan NMR Scanner

**Table 1.** Models of pacemakers and lead systems tested

| | | | |
|---|---|---|---|
| *Pacemaker pulse generators tested in the NMR scanner:* | | | |
| Medtronic: | Xyrel | Biotronic: | Diplos 03, 05 |
| | Versatrax | | Chronos |
| | Activitrax I, II | | Kalos |
| | Spectrax VM, S | | Neos |
| | Spectrax SX, SXT | | Mikros |
| | Enertrax | | Bioguard |
| *Lead systems used for in vitro NMR studies:* | | | |
| Medtronic: | Target tip (uni- or bipolar) | | |
| | 6957/58 and /85 (unipolar) | | |
| Biotronic: | PE 60 (unipolar) | | |

was used. As NMR scanners of different manufacturers function differently, the results obtained canot be transferred to other types without further study.

## Possible Interactions Between Pacemaker and NMR Scanner

For NMR imaging, static magnetic fields (1.5 T, continously), gradient fields (3 mT/min maximum, time-varying), and radio frequencies of 64.26 MHz, 12 kW maximum antenna power level, were tested.

*Static Magnetic Fields.* The main effect was a closure of the pacemaker magnetic reed switch at distances of 4–6 m from the scanner (local field strength = 10 G) and consequently, a switch to an asynchronous pacing mode. We note, however, that in a few pacemaker models, the VVI mode of pacing had persisted during in vitro experiments [7]. It was further observed during in vitro testing that the static magnetic fields induce a torque on the ferrous components of the pacemaker system. Because of the small amount of iron, this torque was negligible. Finally, in a static magnetic field, movement of the pacemaker system generates electric current. There was, however, no evidence during the in vivo testing of any interaction or damage to the pacemaker systems related to static magnetic fields.

*Gradient Fields.* A fast-changing gradient field may induce electric current in a pacemaker system. No effects of such induced electric currents were noticed, either in vitro [7] or in patient studies (myocardial stimulation, pacemaker inhibition during VVI mode, induction of ventricular fibrillation). Nevertheless, the possible influence of induced currents on other parameters of the pacemaker system cannot be neglected. For example, while the activity sensor of a rate-adaptive pacemaker is not influenced by the static magnetic field, it is affected by time-varying gradient fields [11].

*Radio Frequencies.* Radio frequency irradiation may cause warming of the pacemaker system. Theoretically, this could result in thermocoagulation at the electrode site. In our studies, such warming was not observed [9].

## Influence of NMR on Pacing Modes

*VOO Mode.* During NMR, most pacemakers changed to the VOO mode. Resulting asynchronous stimulation could theoretically cause ventricular fibrillation, but this was not observed in our experiments.

*VVI Mode.* The VVI pacemaker mode had been observed to be operational during in vitro experimental investigations [2, 7]. Possibly, this was caused by the magnetic reed switch becoming stuck due to the effects of induced mechanical torsion. During the in vivo testing, 30 of 32 models of pacemaker programmed to the VVI mode changed to VOO during NMR.

*DDD, DDD-R, or VVI-R Modes.* NMR effects on these modes of pacing were not tested. Therefore, these pacing modes should be avoided by appropriate programming of the pacemaker to the VVI mode before NMR imaging. A switch of the programmed mode (VVI) to other modes seems unlikely because of a key word used in the programming code sequence.

*Pacemaker Malfunction (Any Mode).* At least one publication reports pacemaker malfunction (reprogramming, complete pacemaker failure) during in vitro investigations [3]. In our studies, no such malfunction occurred. Pacemaker failure due to malfunction, however, cannot be excluded during NMR scanning. This is especially true for models of pacemakers and lead systems not tested in our studies.

## NMR Scanning Mode for Pacemaker Patients

For our studies [7–10] we used an ECG gated, 2-D multiple slice scanning mode (two to five slices) and a short trigger delay time (0–15 ms). Changes in repetition time or echo time do not influence the pacemaker. The number of slices obtained simultaneously, however, did influence the rate adaptive function of the Activitrax pacemaker [11].

A trigger delay time of 0–15 ms permits the scanning-induced current to cause the myocardium to become refractory, thereby avoiding the possibility of scanning-induced heart stimulation (Fig. 1). With a persistent VVI mode, the pacemaker will still be refractory to inhibition caused by the scanning-induced current. The QRS complex of the ECG or ventricular depolarization following the pacemaker spike has to trigger the NMR scanner. Therefore, a loss of ventricular capture or asystole stops the scanning sequence immediately. Furthermore, an NMR scanning mode triggered by the pacemaker does not cause the myocardium to become refractory after the specified trigger delay time. Yet, scanning-induced current during the trigger delay time, since the myocardium is refractory or partially so, could pace the heart or induce ventricular fibrillation.

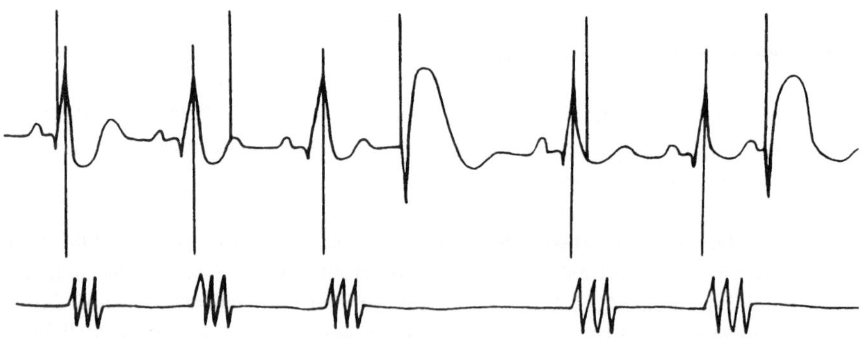

**Fig. 1.** ECG gated NMR scanning (trigger marker within the QRS). NMR scanning time should be limited to the ventricular refractory period

## Recommendations for Pacemaker Programming Before NMR Scanning

*Patients with Adequate Spontaneous Heart Rate.* In the case of adequate spontaneous heart rate or pharmacologically induced (atropine, isoproterenol) heart rate increases, back-up VVI pacing should be performed at a programmed rate of 50 per minute, regardless of pacemaker type. Minimal current and pulse widths should be used to avoid ventricular fibrillation caused by asynchronous pacing. Asynchronous (back-up) pacing is more likely to induce ventricular fibrillation in patients with acid-base, electrolyte, or other physiologic imbalance.

*Pacemaker-Dependent Patients.* In order to ascertain that patients are indeed pacemaker dependent, a sufficient amount of chronotropic drugs should be tested. If the spontaneous rate is still insufficient or there is drug resistance, patients should be overdriven using maximal stimulation (current and pulse width) in the VOO mode. To avoid arrhythmias, the commonly used rate is 100 beats per minute.

*DDD and Rate-Adaptive Pacemakers.* All DDD or rate-adaptive pacemakers should be programmed to the previously described VVI or VOO modes, depending on the patient's intrinsic heart rate.

## Further Requirements for NMR Studies in Pacemaker Patients

Prior to NMR studies, there should be written patient consent for anesthesia and possible revision of the pacemaker system after any NMR imaging. The patient has to be informed that NMR-induced pacemaker failure may lead to the requirement for resuscitation and immediate pacemaker system revision. Further, in order to reduce emotional stress, details about NMR investigation (duration up to 45 min, small tunnel, etc.) should be provided. Finally, the following data have to be documented in the patient's record prior to NMR investigation: spontaneous heart rate, pacemaker status, chest x-ray, response to positive chronotropic drugs, and routine preoperative evaluation for monitored anesthesia care or general anesthesia. In many centers, monitored anesthesia care with only moderate sedation would be used. Even so, preoperative evaluation should be recorded and documented in the patient's chart.

## General Safety Precautions with NMR

Before NMR studies, in vitro tests (in saline solution) of the implanted pacemaker system should have been performed. Emergency equipment must be provided for defibrillation, intubation, and artificial ventilation. The patient must have an empty stomach. Dental prostheses, rings, etc. should be removed. Intravenous (i.v.) access to the patient has to be established from outside the scanner tunnel. Infusion pumps (i.v.) used for chronotropic and other drugs must be able to function in strong NMR fields. While in or near the NMR scanner, the patient should be closely monitored by telemetric ECG transmission, video camera, and an intercom.

If unexpected difficulties do occur, NMR studies should be stopped immediately and the patient removed from the static magnetic field, at least 10 m from the NMR scanner.

## Pacemaker Function and Revision After NMR Studies

After NMR scanning, the pacemaker system should be checked in detail, including an ECG, chest x-ray, magnet test, check for sensing level, pacing threshold test, and test of programming and telemetry function. Optimal pacing parameters have to be reprogrammed for each patient. Additionally, the patient should be observed for at least 24 h in a monitoring unit. If there are any signs of pacemaker malfunction following the NMR studies, the pulse generator may have to be replaced. If sensing levels, pacing thresholds, and lead impedance are adequate, no lead exchange is indicated.

## Conclusions

In general, NMR scanning of pacemaker patients is feasible. Prior to NMR investigation, however, in vitro testing of the implanted pacemaker pulse generator is required. Additionally, safety precautions outlined above should be taken and experienced personnel should be present.

### References


1 Faul DD (1984) Artefakte und Risiken durch Metallimplantate und Herzschrittmacher. Magnetom 10:23–26

2 Chauvin M, Baruthio J, Wolff F et al. (1986) Influences de la resonance magnetique sur les stimulateurs cardiaques implantables. Stimucoeur 14(4):205

3 Erlebacher J, Cahill PT, Panizzo F et al. (1986) Effect of magnetic resonance imaging on DDD pacemakers. Am J Cardiol 57:437–440

4 Fetter J, Aram G, Holmes DR et al. (1984) The effects of nuclear magnetic resonance imagers on external and implantable pulse generators. PACE 7:720–727

5 Holmes DR, Hayes DL, Gray J et al. (1986) The effects of magnetic resonance imaging on implantable pulse generators. PACE 9:360–370

6 Pavlicek W, Geisinger M, Castle L et al. (1983) The effects of nuclear magnetic resonance on patients with cardiac pacemakers. Radiology 147:149–153

7 Iberer F, Justich E, Kapeller J et al. (1987) Untersuchung von Herzschrittmacherträgern mit dem Kernspintomographen – Gefährdung oder Indikation. Acta Chir Austriaca 19(2): 154–155

8 Kapeller J, Iberer F, Justich E et al. (1988) Basic experiments with pacemakers in NMR-tomography equipments. Eur J Clin Invest 18(2):A23

9 Iberer F, Justich E, Stenzl W et al. (1987) Nuclear magnetic resonance imaging of a patient with implanted transvenous pacemaker. Herzschrittmacher 7:196–199

10 Iberer F, Justich E, Stenzl W et al. (1989) Experimental and clinical experience with the magnetic resonance imaging of pacemaker patients. European Symposium on Cardiac Pacing, Stockholm, 1989

11 Iberer F, Justich E, Stenzl W et al. (1987) Behavior of the "Activitrax" pacemaker during nuclear magnetic resonance investigation. 1st International Symposium on Rate Responsive Pacing, Munich, 1987. PACE 10:1215

# Radiation Therapy in Cardiac Pacemaker Patients

M. ANELLI-MONTI, E. POIER, H.E. MÄCHLER AND K. ARIAN-SCHAD

## Introduction

With the increase in cardiac pacemaker implantations, the number of pacemaker patients undergoing radiotherapy is also increasing. At the Department of Surgery, University of Graz, about 600 pacemakers are currently being implanted each year. Approximate 20 patients with pacemakers undergo radiotherapy treatment each year in the Department of Radiotherapy.

Potentially adverse interactions between radiation therapy itself and the implanted pacemaker system can occur for the following reasons: (1) ionizing beams of radiation have direct effects on components of pacemaker systems; (2) electromagnetic fields produced by the linear accelerator may affect sensing function or stimulation mode of the pulse generator.

## Effects of Ionizing Radiation

When discussing effects of radiotherapy, it is necessary to distinguish between treatment volume and irradiated volume. By the former is meant that volume of diseased tissue to which a specified focused dose of irradiation must be applied for a curative effect. While nearby organs and tissues should not be exposed to irradiation, this cannot be totally avoided with percutaneous irradiation, even with a small dose. Therefore, total irradiated volume comprises diseased tissue plus surrounding, nondiseased organs and tissues that are also irradiated.

Interference of irradiation with an implanted pacemaker system is most likely to occur if the pacemaker pulse generator is situated in or near the treatment volume. The result may be either irradiation of the pacemaker pulse generator itself or a reduced dose of irradiation in the treatment volume if the pacemaker system is somehow shielded. Even if the pacemaker is located somewhat peripherally, radiation reaching the pacemaker itself may still be up to 50% of the dose intended for the treatment volume.

Diseases in which radiotherapy might affect pacemakers include: (1) tumors of the breast; (2) carcinoma of the upper lobe of the lungs; (3) systemic lymphomas; (4) ear, nose, throat pathology affecting the supra- or subclavicular region; (5) mesenchymal tumors involving the thoracic wall; and (6) tumors of the skin (basal and spindle cell carcinoma, metastatic melanoma).

Systemic evaluation of the behavior of programmable pacemakers during exposure to irradiation produced by linear accelerators has been investigated by several authors [1–4]. During irradiation exposure of up to 70 Gy (1 Gy = 100 rad), irregular pulse generator output (stimulation) and sensing defects have been reported. However, these results are not applicable to all pacemaker systems because of technical differences between different systems and manufacturers. To evaluate the risks of radiotherapy, separate tests of each system have to be carried out since, in our experience, recommendations supplied by individual manufacturers may be inadequate.

## Effects of Electromagnetic Fields

Electromagnetic fields produced by linear accelerators can interfere with the sensing function of pacemakers by supplying interference signals. Such signals can result in either pacemaker inhibition or a change in stimulation parameters. For example, Venselaar reported complete failure of the stimulation mechanism of a pacemaker while the linear accelerator was being switched on and off [3]. Furthermore, electromagnetic interference (EMI) from the linear accelerator can cause the pacemaker to revert to asynchronous operation, similar to the response to sensed EMI from electrocautery.

## Investigation of the Effects of Radiotherapy on Pacemakers

The foregoing considerations prompted us to carry out in vitro testing of the effects of radiation therapy on different models of pacemakers (Table 1). The pacemakers tested had functioned for periods of up to 2 years and had subsequently been explanted because of infection of the pocket or lead of the pacemaker system. All pacemakers had been checked thoroughly in advance of explantation and had been found to be in good functional order.

First, pacemakers were exposed to the electromagnetic field of a linear accerlator (Saturn 25 CGR, General Electric, Milwaukee, Wisconsin, USA) while positioned just

**Table 1.** Models of pacemakers tested

| Model | Manufacturer | Mode | Polarity | Prog | Tele |
|---|---|---|---|---|---|
| Mikros 02 | Biotronik | VVI | Unipolar | + | + |
| Neos 01 | Biotronik | VVI | Unipolar | + | + |
| Diplos 05M | Biotronik | DDD | Unipolar | + | + |
| Siemens 686 | Siemens | VVI | Unipolar | + | – |
| Spectrac S 5941 | Medtronic | VVI | Unipolar | + | – |
| Spectrac SXT 8423 | Medtronic | VVI | Unipolar | + | + |
| Classix 8438 | Medtronic | VVI | Bipolar | + | + |
| Activitrax 8400 | Medtronic | VVI-R | Bipolar | + | + |
| Activitrax 8403 | Medtronic | VVI-R | Unipolar | + | + |
| Synergist 7070 | Medtronic | DDD-R | Bipolar | + | + |

*Abbrevations:* Mode, ICHD code; Prog, programming function; Tele, Telemetry function; presence (+) or absence (–) of specific function outside of the radiation field. In order to simulate the most unfavorable position for an implanted lead, we arranged a 58 cm lead in a half circle. Pacemaker pulse generator signals (3 mV amplitude, 90 paced pulses per minute) were conveyed by shielded coaxial cables to an oscilloscope display outside the treatment room. Changes in the rate, amplitude, or pattern of stimulation served to verify any pacemaker inhibition or interference during exposure to the electromagnetic field.

Second, effects of direct ionizing radiation were tested using a cobalt irradiator (Theratron 780, Atomic Energy of Canada Ltd., Ottawa). Pacemakers were irradiated in a water tank (37°C) with conventional therapeutic doses of 1 Gy/min up to a maximum of 100 Gy. Again, pacemaker stimuli were continuously displayed on an oscilloscope.

For both types of testing, pacing function was assessed using a pacing system analyzer and an impulse generator. Pacemakers tested were programmed to standard parameters. An external resistance of 470 ohms was used to simulate the patient's impedance. The following pacing parameters were tested: paced pulse rate, pulse amplitude and width, and response of the pacemaker during demand pacing to electromagnetic fields or direct effects of irradiation. Additionally, at intervals of 20 Gy, programming and telemetry function were tested, as also was battery capacity by a magnet test.

## Results of Investigations

*Electromagnetic Field Effects are Produced by the Linear Accelerator.*

Strong electromagnetic interference signals with amplitudes up to 5 V and very short pulse widths (nanoseconds) were observed on the oscilloscope. Electromagnetic interference, however, had no observed effects on pacemaker function.

*Direct Irradiation with Ionizing Radiation*

Eight of ten pacemakers were affected by irradiation (up to 100 Gy) from the cobalt irradiator. The following types of defects were observed:

1. *Complete pacemaker failure.* With two models of pacemakers there was complete failure following exposure to irradiation doses. With the Medtronic Synergist 7070, there was total and irreversible shut-down at 57 Gy. With the Medtronic Spectrax SXT 8423, there was near-complete shut-down, although some irregular pacing pulses persisted at 96 Gy. This reversed after 1 h, but there was still loss of response to a magnet test.

2. *Change of stimulation mode.* With the Biotronik Diplos 05M, initially programmed to the DDD mode, at 88 Gy there was a change from DDD at 70 ppm to VVI at 64 ppm. This change was irreversible despite multiple attempts at reprogramming.

3. *Alteration of stimulation frequency.* With continuous irradiation, in two pacemakers there was a change in stimulation frequency. With the Biotronik Diplos 05M, as noted above, there was an irreversible change in programmed rate from 70 ppm to 64 ppm. With the Medtronic Activitrax 8400, when programmed for rate adaptation

between 56 and 88 ppm, there was a continuous change in the frequency of stimulation during irradiation, except that the programmed rate-adaptive limits (56–88 ppm) were not exceeded. This pattern of response suggests to us that exposure to irradiation may activate the pacemaker's activity sensor, at least with this model of pacemaker.

4. *Increase in pulse width.* The most frequent malfunction of various models of Medtronic pacemakers was an increase in the pulse width. In each individual pacemaker a linear relation between radiation dose and pulse width was found (Fig. 1). Alterations in pulse width were irreversible after completion of irradiation. The first detectable increase in pulse width occurred at 10 Gy for most models of Medtronic pacemakers, which might be considered a warning of sorts for impending pulse width control failure. Similarly, the Biotronik Diplos 05M showed a sudden increase in pulse width at 88 Gy. This occurred as the stimulation mode changed from DDD to VVI (above).

5. *Reduction of pulse amplitude.* Two models of pacemakers showed a reduction in the pulse amplitude during irradiation. The Biotronik Neos 01 device showed a decrease in pulse amplitude from 3.6 to 3.2 V after 100 Gy. This change was entirely reversible 10 days following irradiation. The Biotronik Diplos 05M device showed a 0.4 V decrease in amplitude at 88 Gy.

6. *Demand function.* The demand function was not affected by irradiation in any of the tested pacemaker models. External signals of 3 mV pulse amplitude at 90 ppm safely inhibited all pacemakers.

7. *Programmability.* Irreversible programmability defects occurred in three models of pacemakers (Table 2). For the Medtronic Spectrax SXT and Synergist, from 60 to 80 or 40 to 60 Gy, respectively, programming was no longer possible. This

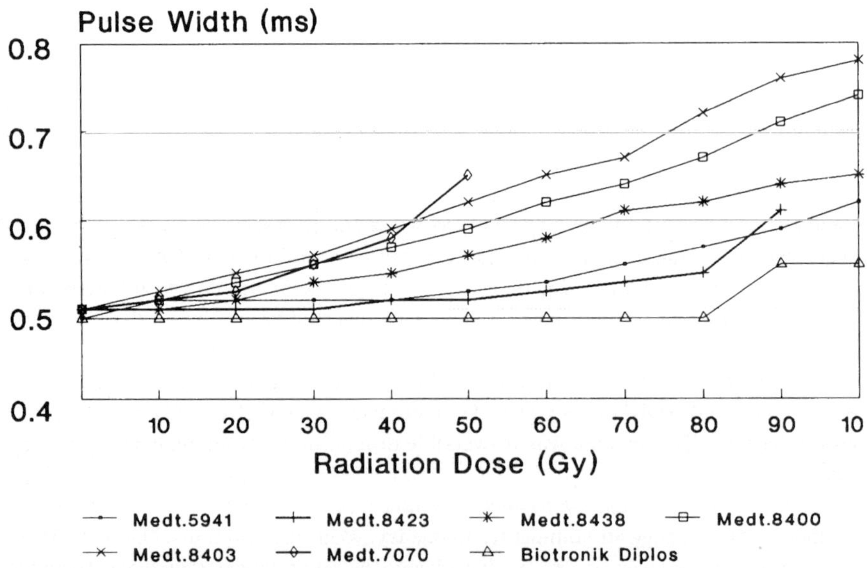


**Fig. 1.** Relation between radiation dose and pulse width (*Medt.*, Medtronic)

**Table 2.** Irradiation-induced defects in programming and telemetry function of pacemakers (the doses cited are those required to alter function)

| Model | Shut-down dose (Gy) | Programming (Gy) | Telemetry (Gy) |
|---|---|---|---|
| Micros 02 | – | – | – |
| Neos 01 | – | – | – |
| Diplos 05M | – | 88 | 88 |
| Siemens 686 | – | – | not available |
| Spectrax S 5941 | – | – | not available |
| Spectrax SXT 8423 | 96 | 68–80 | 60–80 |
| Classic 8438 | – | – | 40–60 |
| Activitrax 8400 | – | – | 80–100 |
| Activitrax 8403 | – | – | 20 |
| Synergist 7070 | 57 | 40–60 | 40–60 |

occurred before total shut-down. For the Biotronik Diplos 05M at 88 Gy following the change from DDD to VVI mode (above), programming was no longer possible.

8. *Telemetry function.* Eight of the ten pacemakers were equipped with telemetry to check actual pacemaker settings. During irradiation, irreversible failure of the telemetric function occurred during exposure to 20–80 Gy (Table 2).

9. *Magnet test.* When an external magnet was applied to pacemakers that still functioned following exposure to irradiation, no change from preset values for frequency or pulse width of resulting asynchronous stimulation was found.

## Conclusions and Recommendations

Two categories of pacemaker malfunction occurred during exposure of pacemakers to irradiation. First, there were functional changes that should pose little risk to the pacemaker patient. Such changes included increases in pulse width, small changes in paced rate, and programming and telemetry function defects. Despite these, however, safe myocardial stimulation parameters were still provided. Any of these functional changes could be diagnosed following radiation therapy using an appropriate pacing system analyzer. Second, there were functional changes in some models of pacemakers that could pose a definite risk to patients. The most important of these was total shut-down, observed in two models. Similar findings have been reported by other authors [1, 3, 4] (Table 3).

As for our specific recommendations, direct exposure of the pulse generator and lead system to irradiation should be avoided. If this is not possible, then the pulse generator should be shielded. Finally, if adequate protection cannot be assured, then it is necessary to carefully monitor the patient for adequate pacemaker function during radiation therapy procedures, including with ECG and some means for detecting heart beats (pulse oximetry, auscultation of heart sounds, direct arterial pressure recording). Additionally, it may be necessary to provide some external means for temporary pacing in case of pacemaker failure during treatment. Finally, pacemaker function should always be checked following treatment. Revision or replacement of the system might be required.

**Table 3.** Defects produced in pacemakers (PM) by irradiation as reported by various authors

| Manufacturer | PM model | Author | Dose (Gy) | Function defects |
|---|---|---|---|---|
| APC | 7131 | V | 100 | Rate |
| APC | 7131 | V | 90 | Rate |
| Biotronik | Nomos | A | 40 | Output |
| Biotronik | Neos | V | 210 | Output |
| Biotronik | Neos | AM | 100 | Pulse amplitude |
| Biotronik | Micros | AM | 100 | – |
| Biotronik | Diplos 05M | AM | 88 | Stimulation mode |
| Cordis | OmniStanicor | V | 590 | Sensing |
| Cordis | OmniStanicor | V | 240 | Sensing |
| Cordis | Sequicor | V | 75 | Output |
| CPI | 505 | A | 10 | Output |
| CPI | 505 | A | 20 | Output |
| CPI | 522 | A | 20 | Output |
| CPI | 622 | V | 23 | Output |
| CPI | 622 | V | 13 | Output |
| CPI | 621 | V | 100 | Sensing |
| Intermedics | Cyberlith | A | 60 | Output |
| Medtronic | 5941 | AM | 100 | Pulse width |
| Medtronic | 8423 | V | 97 | Output |
| Medtronic | 8423 | AM | 96 | Output, telemetry |
| Medtronic | 8438 | AM | 60 | Telemetry, pulse width |
| Medtronic | 8400 | AM | 56–88 | Rate |
| Medtronic | 8400 | AM | 100 | Telemetry, pulse width |
| Medtronic | 8403 | AM | 20 | Telemetry, pulse width |
| Medtronic | 7005 | S | 160 | Output |
| Medtronic | 7070 | AM | 56 | Output |
| Pacesetter | 225 | V | 147 | Rate |
| Pacesetter | 222 | A | 70 | Output |
| Siemens | 668 | V | 750 | Sensing |
| Siemens | 668 | V | 450 | Sensing |
| Siemens | 677 | S | 200 | – |
| Siemens | 678 | S | 200 | – |
| Siemens | 674 | S | 190 | Output |
| Siemens | 686 | AM | 100 | – |
| Siemens | 718 | S | 200 | – |
| Teletronics | OptimaMP | V | 330 | Sensing |
| Teletronics | AutimaII | V | 1500 | – |
| Vitatron | Ceryx3 | V | 120 | Output |
| Vitatron | QuintechTX | V | 57 | Output |
| Vitatron | QuintechDPG | V | 44 | Output |
| Vitatron | QuintechDDD | V | 40 | Output |

Abbreviations for authors: A, Adamec; V, Venselaar; S, Salmi; AM, Anelli-Monti

## References

1 Adamec R, Haeflinger JM, Killisch JP, Niederer J, Jaquet P (1982) Damaging effect of therapeutic radiation on programmable pacemakers. PACE 5:146–148

2 Salmi J, Eskola HJ, Pitkaenen MA, Malmivou JAV (1990) The influence of electromagnetic interference and ionizing radiation on cardiac pacemakers. Strahlenther Onkol 166:153–155

3 Venselaar JLM (1985) The effects of ionizing radiation on eight cardiac pacemakers and the influence of electromagnetic interference from two linear accelerators. Radiother Oncol 3:81–84

4 Venselaar JLM, Kerkoerle HLJM, Vet AJTM (1987) Radiation damage to pacemakers from radiotherapy. PACE 10:538–541

# Extracorporal Shock Wave Lithotripsy in Pacemaker Patients

W. IRNICH, M. LAZICA AND M. GLEISSNER

## Introduction

The noninvasive treatment of nephrolithiasis and, more recently, cholelithiasis with extracorporeal shock wave lithotripsy (ESWL) has gained worldwide acceptance. Between the first successful treatment in 1980 and the end of 1986 were about 30,000 applications in the former Federal Republic of Germany and about 50,000 applications worldwide [1]. In 80% of ESWL interventions, no further surgical treatment has been required.

It can be estimated how often ESWL, with the possible attendant risks, will be performed in pacemaker patients. Approximately 325,000 patients of the 61 million inhabitants of the former Federal Republic of Germany are treated for nephrolithiasis each year. Of these, 50,000 undergo surgery. Yet the annual rate of 8000 ESWLs suggests that this method has not yet reached its full potential. Based on the 1988 figures, the probability of surgical treatment of nephrolithiasis ($8.3 \times 10^{-4}$ per year) in pacemaker patients ($2.5 \times 10^{-3}$ per year) can be estimated at $2.08 \times 10^{-6}$ per year [2]. Consequently, of 61 million inhabitants of the former Federal Republic of Germany, approximately 130 patients with pacemakers can be expected to undergo ESWL each year. While this is a relatively small number of patients, the potential, for complications could be great — hence the present investigation.

## Material and Methods

Thirty-two models of pacemakers from 12 different manufacturers (Table 1) were tested under in vitro conditions to determine whether they could withstand the high ESWL pressure waves and the electromagnetic field caused by the ESWL spark gap without any potential danger to the patient. To this end we produced a holder for the pacemaker that allowed it to be placed in the water of the Dornier lithotriptor in such a way that is could be exposed to shock waves exactly in the second focus of the shock wave ellipsoid. The pacing electrode was arranged in a half circle to approximate the in vivo position. Impulses from the pacemaker were used to trigger the lithotriptor. After 2000 shocks at the maximum voltage setting of 22 kV, pacemaker rate, sensitivity, and output were checked and compared to the data obtained before the test.

**Table 1.** Models of pacemakers tested under in vitro conditions

| Manufacturer | Model | Complication(s) |
|---|---|---|
| 1. Alpha | Alpha 20 | – |
| 2. Biotronik | Axios 04 | – |
| 3. Biotronik | Axios 04 | – |
| 4. Biotronik | Kalos 03–2 | – |
| 5. Biotronik | Neos 01–1 | 1 |
| 6. Cordis | 190A | – |
| 7. Cordis | 190A | – |
| 8. Cordis | 334A | – |
| 9. CPI | 0507 | – |
| 10. CPI | 0523 | – |
| 11. Siemens-Elema | 668 | – |
| 12. Siemens-Elema | 674 | – |
| 13. Siemens-Elema | MP688 | – |
| 14. Intermedics | 253–05 | – |
| 15. Intermedics | 253–07 | – |
| 16. Medtronic | 5985 | 2 |
| 17. Medtronic | 5985 | – |
| 18. Medtronic | 5995 | – |
| 19. Medtronic | 8400 | 3 |
| 20. Medtronic | 8403 | 4 |
| 21. Medtronic | 8423 | – |
| 22. Osypka | Acculith 51 | – |
| 23. Pacesetter | 221A | – |
| 24. Pacesetter | 241 | – |
| 25. Precimed | Precilith 210 | – |
| 26. Precimed | Precilith 215 | – |
| 27. Telectronics | 183 | – |
| 28. Telectronics | Optima-MP | – |
| 29. Vitatron | P4122 | 5 |
| 30. Vitatron | P4122 | 5 |
| 31. Vitatron | P4122 | 5 |
| 32. Vitatron | Ceryx 6 | – |

*Complications:*
1. After 400 shocks irregular rate and decrease in rate from 60 to 54 ppm
2. Prior to the shock application there were rate irregularities, then total malfunction with ESWL
3. End of service (EOS) rate, insulation defect between battery and pulse generator can, piezolectric crystal sensor defect following 3000 shocks
4. EOS readout; able to reprogram
5. Rate abnormalities up to 94 ppm (not magnetic interference rate)

After in vitro testing of the first 15 models of pacemakers without serious interference and no defects following exposure to ESWL [3], ESWL was performed in 14 pacemaker patients with "safe" units. The following precautionary measures were observed:

1. The model of pacemaker in question was shown not to be affected (i.e., to be "safe") under in vitro testing conditions.

2. Temporary pacing electrodes were placed as a prophylactic measure in pacemaker-dependent patients.
3. Both a cardiologist and a defibrillator with an external temporary pulse generator were readily available during the ESWL treatment.

The 14 patients treated had one of the following indications for pacing: atrioventricular block (6), sick sinus syndrome (5), sinuatrial block (2), and symptomatic sinus bradycardia (1).

## Results

### *In Vitro Testing*

Pressures in the second focus of the ESWL ellipsoid reached up to 43MPa (which is 430 bar or atmospheres) over a period of 5 μs [4]. At a distance of 5 mm, pressures were 80%–90% of these values, while at 1 cm they fell to about 40%. These results demonstrate the enormous focused power of ESWL shock waves, which surprisingly had little effect on pacemakers tested (Table 1). Nevertheless, of the 32 systems tested, seven units were affected either by the pressure waves or by the electromagnetic field of the lithotriptor. Principal adverse effects are listed as "complications" beneath Table 1. Some of these are described in more detail below.

The Medtronic pacemaker with complication 2 was totally disabled by the ESWL test. However, retrospective analysis of this particular unit's function prior to testing revealed rate abnormalities. Consequently, it is difficult to determine to what extent the total system failure with ESWL was caused by ESWL, and to what extent by the preexisting defect.

The rate responsive pacemakers with complications 3 and 4 showed a rate reduction which indicates approaching power source depletion (end-of-service readout, EOS). However, both pacemakers could be reprogrammed. In the case of the bipolar pacemaker with complication 3, an insulation defect occurred between the battery and the can of the generator. The resulting contact between the different electrode and the can caused a short circuit, and resultant switching to the EOS rate. After an additional 1000 shocks (total of 3000 shocks), a non-reprogrammable defect in the sensor circuit (piezoelectric crystal) also occurred.

Finally, the pacemaker with complication 5 showed rate abnormalities during ESWL testing, with rates up to 94 ppm. Rates did not correspond to the magnetic interference rate, as we originally assumed. Following completion of the test, however, this pacemaker was completely functional.

### *ESWL in Patients with Pacemakers*

Two of the 14 patients treated with ESWL showed unexpected results. In one patient, heart rate increased from 70 to 80 beats per minute during the ESWL treatment. This rate increase was due to supraventricular extrasystoles. We believe ESWL shock waves transmitted to the thorax and heart were responsible for this phenomenon. Post facto examination of patient's ECGs before lithotripsy, however, showed a tendency to supraventricular extrasystoles. Nevertheless, these became more frequent during ESWL. Walts and Atlee [10] also reported short runs of supraventricular tachycardia in two patients undergoing ESWL.

In a second patient, an intermittent sensing defect appeared subsequent to ESWL. Following pacemaker exchange after ESWL, there were no apparent abnormalities involving either the removed pulse generator or the leads. We believe that a previously suspected (but never documented) faulty electrode contact became manifest during ESWL, possibly due to localized pressure effects of the ESWL shock waves.

During lithotripsy treatment in two patients, a nonsychronized ESWL shock trigger (to ECG R wave or pacemaker stimulus artifact) was deliberately used to provoke possible untoward effects on pacemaker sensing function. Results of this additional testing were remarkable for two reasons. First, neither of the two pacemakers tested was influenced by the electric or magnetic fields produced by ESWL spark discharge. Second, both patients manifested ventricular extrasystoles. These occurred mainly at the end of the T wave. We speculate that ventricular extrasystoles were caused by nonsynchronized ESWL shocks during the vulnerable period of the ventricles. Despite nonsynchronized ESWL shocks or ventricular extrasystoles, however, the pacemakers in both patients continued to sense R waves and not artifacts produced by ESWL shocks.

## Discussion

Apparently, modern demand pacemakers are sufficiently robust to withstand the high pressure shock waves generated during lithotripsy. In addition, electromagnetic fields caused by the ignition spark would seem to have no important adverse effects on the pacemaker systems tested. The reason for the latter might be that electromagnetic fields, even though they are induced by up to 120 V, are filtered out by sensing amplifiers because their pulse durations are in the microsecond range. Furthermore, induced electromagnetic artifacts fall into the refractory period of demand pacemakers during normal ESWL treatment. The delay between the synchronized heart (ECG) signal and activation of the ESWL spark gap ranges between 120 and 160 ms, at least with the lithotriptor used in our investigation. Finally concerning this investigation, we note that tolerable rate changes in the pacemaker with complication 5 (Table 1) occurred only during in vitro testing and not in patients.

A literature search (journal PACE) revealed similar findings by others working in the same field (Table 2). An analysis of data from the 32 pacemakers we tested and 112 similarly tested pacemakers from the literature indicated that 6 of 144 pacemakers (4.2%) failed when exposed to ESWL. It is apparent that pacemakers with a piezoelectric crystal sensor are most susceptible to failure. Consequently, patients with these types of pacemakers require careful follow up following any ESWL.

Based on our results, as well of those of other authors [5–9], we believe that ESWL can be tolerated by most pacemaker patients. We say this, however, with certain reservations:

**Table 2.** ESWL effects on pacemakers. Result of in vitro testing by other authors

| Authors | Effects of ESWL treatment |
|---|---|
| Cooper et al. [5] | 18 – 22 kV ESWL, 15 pacemakers, in focus of shock wave ellipsoid, 1300 shocks, two pacemaker failures |
| Fetter et al. [6] | Miscellaneous (Medtronic) VVI and DDD pacemakers placed on the skin, intermittent QRS synchronizing defects |
| Garza et al. [7] | 9 pacemaker models from 4 manufacturers:<br>1. 4 cm from focus, 100–200 shocks, one pacemaker unhibited<br>2. Placed on skin, up to 600 shocks, no failures<br>3. In focus, 200 shocks, all pacemakers showed synchronization defects, two with mechanical defects |
| Langberg et al. [8] | 22 pacemakers (16 models from 8 manufacturers), 5 cm from focus, one unit reverted to magnet rate, half had synchronization defects |
| Markewitz et al. [9] | 66 pacemakers (50 models from 11 manufacturers), in focus, up to 3000 shocks, 4 units reverted to magnet rate, 8 had synchronization defects |

1. Pacemakers not tested could react differently when exposed to ESWL. For this reason an unknown pacemaker should be tested under in vitro conditions similar to those described above before a patient with such a pacemaker is subjected to ESWL.
2. In pacemaker systems with inherent mechanical defects (e.g., loose contacts, cold-soldered joints, weak contacts) further breakdown could be provoked by ESWL pressure waves. Therefore, institution of at least a back-up temporary pacing capability is advised in pacemaker-dependent patients.
3. Previous reports suggest that inappropriate inhibition or triggering of pacemaker output by the ESWL discharge spark cannot be excluded if the lithotriptor works in an asynchronous mode [6–9], even though this did not happen with the pacemakers tested in this study. For this reason, the lithotriptor should always be triggered by the ventricular depolarization (QRS) signal. If the lithotriptor is synchronized with the pacemaker spike (which was not the case in our study), it is possible with a dual chamber pacemaker (e.g., DDD mode) that the atrial impulse could trigger the lithotriptor. Since the ESWL shock wave output is delayed by up to 160 ms, this could in theory be detected by the ventricular sensing amplifier, and the ventricular stimulus inhibited. Thus, during ESWL treatment, a DDD pacing system should be programmed to the VVI mode.
4. During ESWL, there should always be an experienced cardiologist readily available, one who could intervene quickly in the rare event of pacemaker failure.
5. Any rate-responsive pacemakers should be programmed in their non-rate-sensing mode to avoid rate alterations with ESWL.

6. All pacemaker systems should be checked immediately following ESWL treatment for proper function.

## Summary and Conclusions

The noninvasive treatment of nephrolithiasis, and more recently cholelithiasis, with ESWL has gained world wide acceptance. The numbers of pacemaker patients who might undergo ESWL can be estimated. This investigation attempted to ascertain whether ESWL can be safely performed in pacemaker patients. Both in vitro and in vivo methods were tested. First, 32 models of pacemakers from 12 different manufacturers were exposed to 2000 shock waves in the focus of the ESWL ellipsoid. Second, 14 pacemaker patients underwent ESWL after successful testing of their model of pacemaker under in vitro conditions (i.e., under these conditions the model in question had been shown to be unaffected by ESWL). During in vitro testing, one out of 32 pacemakers tested failed completely, five pacemakers showed rate changes, and one pacemaker had insulation and sensor defects after 3000 shocks. Of 14 patients with pacemakers who underwent ESWL, in one there was a rate increase from 70 to 80 ppm and in another the demand function failed intermittently. A literature search revealed comparable results. In conclusion, we believe that ESWL can be performed safely in pacemaker patients, provided adequate precautionary measures are taken.

## References

1 Schmiedt E (1984) Die experimentelle Entwicklung der ESWL, Symposium anläßlich der 1000. ESWL-Behandlung, 17. Feb. 1984

2 Irnich W, Batz L (1989) Jahresbericht 1988 des Zentralregisters Herzschrittmacher. Herzschrittmacher 9:192–197

3 Lazica M, Gleissner M, Irnich W, Albrecht KF (1985) Erste Untersuchungen und Erfahrungen mit der ESWL-Behandlung der Schrittmacherpatienten. Verh Dtsch Ges Urol 36:140–145

4 Lazica M (1987) Experimentelle Untersuchungen an Schrittmachern unter den Bedingungen der extrakorporalen Stoßwellenlithotripsie. Dissertation, Medical faculty, University of Cologne

5 Cooper D, Wilkoff B, Masterson M et al. (1988) Effects of extracorporeal shock wave lithotripsy on cardiae pacemakers and its safety in patients with implanted cardiac pacemakers. PACE 11:1607–1616

6 Fetter J, Hayes D, Aram G et al. (1987) Electrohydraulic shock wave lithotripsy effects on cardiac pulse generators. PACE 10:674 (abstract)

7 Garza J, Tansey M, Florio J, Messenger J (1987) The effect of extracorporeal shockwave lithotripsy on implanted cardiac pacemakers. PACE 10:675 (abstract)

8 Langberg J, Arber J, Thuroff JW, Griffin JC (1987) The effects of extracorporeal shock wave lithotripsy on pacemaker function. PACE 10:1142–1146

9 Markewitz A, Weber W, Wildgans H, Winhold C (1987) Does extracorporeal shock wave lithotripsy affect pacemaker function? PACE 10:711 (abstract)

10 Walts LF, Atleee JR (1986) Supraventricular tachycardia associated with extracorporeal shock wave lithotripsy. Anesthesiology 65:521–523

# Pacemaker Malfunction: The European Legal Perspective

P. SCHICK AND W. POSCH

## Penal Sanctions

### *Theoretical Framework*

Pacemaker technology has advanced enormously during the last decade. Today, pacemakers are generally implanted in the course of a relatively benign surgical procedure performed under local anesthesia. The pacemaker itself is not much larger than a small match box. Further, currently implanted devices are relatively inconspicuous and patient oriented, and provide a high degree of accuracy and reliability.

The implantation of a pacemaker qualifies as curative operation or treatment. According to the doctrine of recent Austrian penal law such treatment, if medically indicated, correctly performed, and serving a therapeutic purpose, does not constitute a personal injury as prohibited by the Penal Code.

Medical activity is evaluated by the general standards of negligence. These are provided for by §6 StGB (Austrian Penal Code). The so-called medical doctor's privilege [§88 (2) no. 2 StGB], which grants a medical practitioner exemption from punishment if he is responsible only for simple negligence and if the injurious result does not surpass 2 weeks of illness or disability, has no practical importance at all. Originally, §88 (2) no. 2 StGB was intended to demonstrate the legislator's concern at the high risks that are involved in medical practice. However, "high risks" is subject to interpretation as the code refers to "extraordinarily dangerous circumstances" (§81 no. 1 StGB), as well as to "high probability of the occurrence of injury". If either of these exist, however, the granting of the so-called medical doctor's privilege is excluded. It is clear from the wording of §88 StGB, that only a "simple personal injury, not a qualified one", may give rise to a medical doctor's privilege.

In most cases, the practitioner's acts are "unconsciously negligent". This means that the practitioner fails to provide such care as required of him under the circumstances, as well as such care as may reasonably be expected of him based on his mental and physical capacities [§6 (1) StGB]. In contrast, "wanton negligence" [§6 (2) StGB] requires that the offending practitioner considers the prohibited result possible, but does not desire this result. For example, he assumes he will be able to avoid any risks associated with his activities. Such situations of "wanton negligence" may occur in cases of therapeutic and nontherapeutic experiments, as might currently be the case with respect to implantation of an artificial heart.

The objective standard of a practitioner's duty of care follows to a lesser degree from relevant statutory provisions (Medical Doctor's Act, Hospital Act, etc.). More important are the rules of the medical profession representing the actual state of the art, as well as the degree of care a prudent and upright person, being a member of the same profession, would provide in the offender's position in order to prevent the occurrence of injury. The cautious and judicious "model" practitioner, who adheres to the values of his profession, will, in addition to providing regular care, be inclined to exhaust all means of reducing risks attendant upon medical procedures performed by him.

The subjective violation of due care depends on the offender's physical and mental capacity as well as his ability to behave lawfully. Whether subjective violation of due care can be found depends on examination of the offender's particular position. The higher his educational qualification and professional experience, the higher will be the level of care expected from the offender. If the offending practitioner, knowingly aware of his own limitations, incurs a risk, he still may not be blamed for any subsequent treatment failure, but only for initiating a potentially injurious procedure or activity.

Another important aspect of the medical due care concept that must be considered in order to establish negligence is the fact that medical services are usually rendered by a team of physicians. Every member of the team is liable under the threat of criminal sanction for the performance of his specific duties as part of that team. He is entitled, however, to rely on every other team member's careful performance of his particular duty of care. Each member's own duty of care is limited by the so-called reliance rule. The validity of this rule is limited, however. If the behavior of the person to whom reliance should be addressed is ambiguous and obscure, the "reliance rule" provides no defense.

### *Penal Law Theory Applied to Pacemaker Failures*

In the following sections, we turn from consideration of theoretical concepts to practical aspects. We now deal with the question of the consequences provided for by Austrian penal law if risks attendant upon the manufacture or implantation of pacemakers, or related treatment in pacemaker patients, materialize in connection with the use of pacemakers in patients.

*Manufacture and Distribution of Pacemakers.* Criminal liability is always dependent on establishing fault. Therefore, defects in a pacemaker system that cause injury to the patient will be sanctioned by criminal law only in rare cases. In contrast to the fault-based criminal liability, liability for injury to a patient caused by a defective product has only recently been introduced in civil tort law by the Product Liability Act of 21 January 1988 (Official Journal No. 99/1988), following the model of the EEC Directive of 27 July 1985.

*Selection and Implantation of a Pacemaker.* It may be assumed that products reaching the market have undergone detailed clinical testing and conform with the state of the art of medical techniques. Pacemakers must be officially approved by the state authority. As a rule, the implanting surgeon may rely on faultless functioning of the pacemaker device based on its certification by the public authority, unless his own superficial inspection reveals a defect (physical or functional) of that device. The law does not require that a detailed check be made of each pacemaker unit to be implanted by some technical (engineering) official of the hospital. However, if the implanting physician has doubt as to the functioning of a particular brand of pacemaker, he may be well advised to consult the engineering official of his hospital.

Many different models of pacemakers are distributed in Austria and elsewhere, each designed to serve different functions to meet specific medical indications. If, for example, a surgeon implants a rather simple pacemaker (e.g., ventricular asynchronous) instead of a more sophisticated one (e.g., atrial triggered) in a patient suffering from sinus node incompetence, but with intact AV conduction, and the patient suffers symptoms of cardiac insufficiency, such an occurrence could qualify as carelessness on the part of the implanting physician. This could result in criminal sanctions. The same principles apply if there are technical deficiencies in the pacemaker implantation procedure on the part of the implanting physician.

*Postoperative Treatment and Follow-up.* Pacemaker manufacturers publish "pacemaker brochures" which provide information and advice to patients with pacemakers. These directives must be given and reasonably explained to the patient by the implanting physician after a successful pacemaker implantation. Depending on the circumstances of a particular case, the implanting physician may be obligated to provide additional oral or written advice to the patient.

Regular pacemaker follow-up checks should be performed as a matter of routine. In particular, towards the end of the useful life of the pacemaker (approximately 6—8 years), pacemaker function must be ascertained frequently and with utmost care. If any malfunction of the device is discovered or suspected, the pacemaker must be repaired or exchanged.

Finally, if, following pacemaker implantation, the patient develops a new disease or condition requiring treatment, the responsible implanting physician has the duty to inform any other colleague involved in the medical or surgical treatment (or diagnosis) of the patient about special risk(s) occasioned by the presence of the pacemaker, as well as the reason for its implantation, its type, and its construction.

*Subsequent Treatment of Pacemaker Patients.* The increasing use of complex technology in the construction of pacemakers makes it necessary for physicians involved with the care of pacemaker patients to have at least basic knowledge of the design and function of electronic cardiac pacemakers. In the same way that the physician is expected to be knowledgeable concerning the potential side effects or adverse effects of pharmaceuticals he prescribes, he must also be aware of potential side-effects or adverse effects of pacemakers, as well as dangers of malfunction of such devices.

Only if the implanting physician has full knowledge of the design and intended function of the pacemaker system he prescribes for his patient will he be able to recognize the potentially dangerous impact of pacemaker malfunction upon the health of his patient. The nonimplanting physician does not require such detailed knowledge, but he has the duty to consult an expert when in doubt concerning management or treatment of a referred pacemaker patient. If a physician is unable to recognize dangers to the patient's health posed by the interaction of his treatment with a pacemaker, perhaps because he does not understand how the pacemaker works or for lack of relevant information, he may be liable for any resulting personal injury to the patient due to his negligence. This would be the case, for example, if the implanting physician did not carefully read the instructions for use attached to the pacemaker by the manufacturer, or if the physician (e.g., surgeon, anesthesiologist, radiologist) did not consult a pacemaker expert prior to treatment which could harm the pacemaker patient.

If the physician responsible for treatment and follow-up of a pacemaker patient attempts to obtain all necessary information, but is still uncertain as to the effect of his treatment (e.g., radiation therapy) on pacemaker function, he still has the duty to the patient of finding some means of reducing the remaining risk of malfunction. Such means might include reprogramming of the pacemaker, disabling its function for a short period of time and application of additional shielding, as well as provision for back-up temporary pacing, electroversion of the heart, chronotropic drugs, or intensive medical care should the pacemaker malfunction as a result of his treatment.

If obstacles prevent the consulting physician from taking indicated risk-minimizing measures, he should not engage in treatment of a pacemaker patient. If he does so, he could be responsible for any adverse outcome to the patient as a result of his treatment. If, however, there would have been greater immediate danger to the patient as a result of withholding treatment, it may be necessary for him to provide this treatment despite the danger of causing pacemaker malfunction. Only in this circumstance can the consulting physician be held blameless.

Therefore, physicians, patients, and the courts increasingly find themselves in a vicious circle. As current medical practice, seemingly mostly for the benefit of patients but also with financial incentives for the physician, becomes more and more dependent on technical innovations, the objective and subjective standards of care which the law imposes on the medical profession may become even more restrictive.

## Civil Liability

### *Manufacturer's Liability*

If pacemaker malfunction results in personal injury or death, there is the question of whether the victim may bring a claim in tort and, if so, against whom. In most EEC member countries and Scandinavian countries, new product liability statutes have recently been or will be enacted pursuant to the EEC Directive of 27 July 1985 (O.J. L 210). The new Austrian product liability law (PHG), which is highly consonant with provisions of the EEC Directive, came into force on 1 July 1988 (O.J. = BGBl. 1988/89). This new statute provides for a cause of action against the manufacturer, importer, or distributor of a defective pacemaker that causes injury or death to a patient.

Liability is imposed on manufacturers, on importers, and (within specific limits) also on distributors of defective products. As pacemakers are movable goods, they are covered by the product liability act's definition of "product" (§4 PHG). The liability under the product liability act is imposed irrespective of whether a negligent behavior is involved or not. All European product liability statutes now follow the American model of strict liability. Between American and European product liability laws, including those of Austria, there remain significant differences, however, in particular with regard to the recoverable amounts of damage.

Thus pacemaker manufacturers and importers cannot escape liability simply by proving that they are not to blame for negligence caused by themselves or their employees. Distributors of pacemakers, however, may only become liable if they sell an anonymous product and are unable to provide information within a reasonable time period about the identity of the manufacturer, importer, or wholesaler from whom they obtained the product. As pacemakers are proprietary items, a self- or hospital-employed physician may not become liable just because he selected and implanted a defective pacemaker. This is especially so if the defectiveness of the device was not immediately apparent upon superficial inspection.

Pursuant to the new product liability rules, only the manufacturer or importer of a pacemaker can be held strictly liable for any type of personal injury resulting from a defective pacemaker. Under Austrian law, strict liability also extends to pain and suffering. Liability under the new product liability act is also imposed on manufacturers of component pacemaker parts. Therefore, it is possible that the manufacturer or importer of a defective power source (battery) used in a pacemaker could also be held liable together with the manufacturer or importer of the entire pacemaker system.

Civil liability is dependent on how defective the pacemaker is. The test for defectiveness is regulated by §5 PHG. Pursuant to this provision with some reservations for special mitigating circumstances, a product may be found defective if it does not meet the safety expectations of an average informed user. In the case of a highly sensitive and technical product, malfunction of which could result in severe personal injury, the consumer (patient) is entitled to an augmented standard of safety expectation. This says, in effect, that the patient may rely on the correct functioning of the pacemaker during its entire useful life, as explained to him by the manufacturer or physician performing pacemaker treatment.

The manufacturer has to provide precise information to the implanting physician about requirements for implantation and the characteristics of the pacemaker. However, since the pacemaker must be implanted by a physician, the manufacturer must also rely on the expertise of the implanting physician. The manufacturer has an added duty to warn pacemaker patients in no uncertain terms of potential harmful effects of pacemakers or interactions that could result in malfunction. The latter could include electromagnetic interference, effects of ionizing radiation, etc. The manufacturer must also provide instructions both to the patient and to his implanting physician for reducing such risk. Since the burden of proof is imposed on the manufacturer, he will have to be sure that these instructions are definitely conveyed to pacemaker patients and implanting physicians. Only in this way can the legitimate safety expectations of the consumer be satisfied.

If the manufacturer has expressed or provided detailed warnings and instructions, but the product fails to conform to the relevant state of the art, the manufacturer may still be held responsible for injury to the patient. Therefore, if it is technically possible to produce pacemakers that are compatible with electromagnetic fields, the manufacturer has the duty and responsibility to do so. It is not sufficient, then, for the manufacturer simply to warn of dangers of exposure of pacemakers to magnetic fields.

Under the new product liability law the victim of a defective pacemaker has to prove that the product was already defective at the time it was released by the manufacturer or importer. Such proof may be difficult under the circumstances. However, if there is evidence of a defective pacemaker and it can be established that this was the cause of injury or death, the manufacturer can escape civil liability only by providing that the defect was caused by mandated compliance with legal sanctions or administrative codes. To our knowledge, no such legal sanctions or administrative codes currently exist in Austria. Another defense available to the manufacturer or importer is to prove that the pacemaker could not have been discovered as defective at the time the pacemaker was first marketed.

Provisions of the product liability act of 1988 state that liability for claims brought by the victim of a defective product is always joint and several. Additionally, payment for damages may be the shared responsibility of several parties. Finally, claims must be brought within 3 years after the victim learned of his injury and received information about the identity of the responsible manufacturer or importer. The absolute limit for claims is 10 years from the date the manufacturer or importer first put the defective product into circulation.

### *Physician's Liability*

In addition to liability of the pacemaker manufacturer, importer, or distributor, the physician selecting a particular pacemaker for his patient may also be held liable. However, such liability is not based on provisions of the product liability act of 1988. If, for example, the physician was negligent in that he prescribed or implanted the wrong type of pacemaker, he will be held liable on the basis of the general rules of liability. It is not sufficient for the responsible physician to claim that he selected a less costly but ineffective or unsafe pacemaker system in the interest of reducing costs.

Concerning the technical knowledge and expertise expected of implanting physicians, it is not expected that a medical doctor can be an expert in biomedical technology or engineering. According to §1 of the Austrian Medical Doctors Act, the medical profession includes "every kind of activity based on medicoscientific knowledge that can be applied directly to human beings". Therefore, it may be reasonably expected of a physician specializing in pacemaker implantations that he has the knowledge to program such devices and to recognize deficiencies of various models of pacemakers. If he lacks such knowledge or ability, he may become liable under the aggregated standards of collective liability established for experts by §1299 and 1300 of the Austrian Civil Code. In particular, the doctor implanting a pacemaker system is responsible for adhering to instructions and recommendations provided to him by the manufacturer, as well as for selection of the pacemaker system to be implanted. He is also responsible for conveying correct information to the patient with regard to potential complications due to the pacemaker.

It is evident that the responsible pacemaker physician can be held liable for any adverse outcome to the patient which results from his negligence. This could be due to selection of an improper device, incorrect operative management, or inadequate management following pacemaker implantation. Since the burden of proof of no fault is the responsibility of the physician, he is well advised to adequately document all pertinent information concerning indications for pacing, device selection, implantation procedure, programming information, and pacemaker follow-up.

# Indications for Pacing: The Cardiologist's Perspective

W. KLEIN AND B. ROTMAN

This discussion of indications for implantation of cardiac pacemakers is subdivided into three parts. First, we consider arrhythmias and disturbances of conduction for which pacing therapy is indicated. Second, diagnostic tests and procedures which are used prior to pacemaker implantation are discussed. Finally, we address the issue of which pacemaker should be chosen for a particular pacing indication.

## Indications for Pacemakers

Major indications for pacing at our institution are bradycardia with or without associated tachyarrhythmias due to sinus node dysfunction and atrioventricular block. More than half of the patients receiving pacemakers will have sinus node dysfunction. The latter can be intrinsic dysfunction caused by atrial disorders or an extrinsic form due to defective neurogenic autonomic nervous system regulation. Both forms of sinus node dysfunction can be the cause of vertigo, syncope, dizziness, malaise, or heart failure. Sudden cardiac death, however, is not commonly associated with these disorders.

### *Intrinsic Sinus Node Dysfunction*

The intrinsic form of sinus node dysfunction is more commonly referred to as the sick sinus syndrome and represents an atrial disorder. The ECG can show sinus bradycardia, sinus pauses or arrest, and sinoatrial exit block. Any of these may be associated with alternating periods of tachycardia, the so-called bradycardia-tachycardia syndrome. There can also be a bradycardic form of atrial fibrillation or flutter associated with sinus node dysfunction.

In the case of bradyarrhythmias, a pacemaker is only indicated if the patient is symptomatic and the symptoms can be attributed to the bradyarrhythmias. In the absence of symptoms no further investigation or therapy is necessary. Only a small number of patients with bradyarrhythmias due to sinus node dysfunction have symptoms, and only these patients require a pacemaker.

*Atrioventricular Block*

In contrast, high degree AV block usually constitutes a very clear indication for the implantation of a pacemaker, since it usually produces symptomatic bradycardia. AV block is most often due to longstanding systemic hypertension, cardiosclerosis, or primary disorders of the conduction system. More rarely it is caused by coronary insufficiency or myocarditis. Recently it has been said that infrahisian AV block could be caused by an immunological process [1].

In May of 1984, the North American Society of Pacing and Electrophysiology issued the following guidelines for pacemaker insertion [2]:

| | |
|---|---|
| Class I indication: | general agreement as to a clear indication for a pacemaker |
| Class II indication: | pacemakers are often used but the indication is a matter of some dispute |
| Class III indication: | general agreement that a pacemaker is not indicated |

A class I indication for the implantation of a cardiac pacemaker in a patient with chronic or intermittent second or third degree AV block or atrial fibrillation with the same, would be one or more of the symptoms or findings listed in Table 1. Such patients following pacemaker implantation can except an improvement in 5-years survival of from 30% to 60% [3].

Following acute myocardial infarction, a permanent pacemaker is indicated only for persistent AV block at the time of discharge from the hospital. However, it is a matter of dispute (class II indication) as to whether a permanent pacemaker should be implanted in a patient with persistent first degree AV block and new bundle branch block following acute myocardial infarction. Also not agreed to as an indication for permanent pacing is transient AV block or bundle branch block following acute myocardial infarction.

Concerning class III indications, it has been discussed whether bifascicular block (left anterior or posterior fascicular with right bundle branch block, or left bundle branch block) constitutes an indication for permanent pacing. Several studies and especially those by Dhingra et al. [4] and McAnulty et al. [5, 6], have suggested that only 10% of patients with bifascicular block develop complete heart block within 7 years. Sudden cardiac death due to bradyarrhythmias in these patients is very unusual. Rather the high mortality (50%–60%) within the first 7 years is caused by the cardiac disorder underlying the bradyarrhythmias or by tachyarrhythmias. Thus, the indication for a permanent pacemaker in patients with chronic bifascicular block is only given

**Table 1.** Class I indications for a pacemaker in patients with chronic or intermittent second or third degree AV block

1. Symptomatic bradycardia
2. Congestive heart failure
3. Ventricular arrhythmias associated with heart block that require treatment
4. Cardiac arrest >3 s or escape rhythm < 40 bpm in asymptomatic patients
5. Symptoms of dizziness or drowsiness which respond to temporary pacing

for those patients with symptomatic bradycardia and intermittent second or third degree AV block. Bifascicular block without intermittent high degree AV block or symptoms attributable to bradycardia does not constitute an indication for permanent pacing.

Expanding on the argument for permanent pacing with bifascicular block or intermittent second (type II or Mobitz) or third degree AV block, it is to be pointed out that such a block is usually due to degenerative changes within the conduction system below the AV node. Type I (Wenckebach) second degree AV block, on the other hand, is more likely to result from depressant effects of drugs at the AV node. Therefore, reversal is by removal of the offending drug(s) or substitution by one less likely to prolong AV node conduction time or refractoriness. Only if medications cannot be removed or effective substitutions made should consideration be guided to permanent pacing, and then only if the patient has symptomatic bradycardia due to second degree AV block (type I).

Other factors that could affect the decision to implant a permanent pacemaker in patients with atrioventricular block are listed in Table 2.

**Table 2.** Further factors which could influence the decision to implant a permanent pacemaker

1. The patient's physical condition, especially when life expectancy is short
2. The patient must drive in public or operate hazardous machinery
3. Limited access to or for removal from a medical facility
4. Requirement for medication with negative chronotropic or dromotropic actions
5. The presence of slow escape rhythms
6. Associated cardiac disease
7. The patient's personal preferences, life-style, etc.

*Hypersensitive Carotid Sinus Syndrome*

A permanent pacemaker may be indicated in patients with a history of syncopal episodes in whom symptoms can be provoked by external stimulation of the carotid sinus or in whom asystole >3 s can be produced by carotid sinus massage. However, such stimulation (e.g., with tilt testing) or carotid sinus massage should be performed in the absence of medication known to inhibit the carotid sinus reflex (baroreflex). The hypersensitive carotid sinus syndrome can be of the inhibitory (bradycardia) or vasodepressor (vasodilation) type. Pacing is not indicated for the forms without symptoms attributable to bradycardia; that is, pacing is not effective treatment for the vasodepressor type of carotid sinus syndrome.

## Diagnostic Tests and Procedures

*Sinus Node Dysfunction*

Holter monitoring has shown that daytime rates of 37–65 beats per minute and cardiac asystole up to 1.7s, or nighttime rates of 33–55 beats per minute and asystole up to 2 s are tolerated. For pacing to be indicated, the 24-hour ECG must show rates below 30 beats per minute with sick sinus syndrome, as well as periods of asystole >3 s. An exercise test provides an excellent diagnostic tool for documenting chronotropic imcompetence. A pacemaker is indicated if, with stress testing, the sinus rate does not reach 100 beats per minute or there is an increase in sinoatrial or AV block with exercise. Furthermore, pharmacological measures may be used (atropine or β-adrenergic agonists) to assess chronotropic competence. One such test is the i.v. administration of 0.02 mg/kg atropine. If the heart rate does not increase at least 25% above its initial value, a pacemaker may be indicated. Isoproterenol is also used for this purpose.

Electrophysiological testing, including His bundle ECG recording, is sometimes used to test asymptomatic patients with suggestive signs of the sick sinus syndrome on 24-hour ECG recordings. With rapid stimulation of the atrium, it is possible to determine the sinus node recovery time (SRT) or SRT corrected for spontaneous heart rate (CSRT). A value for CSRT >450 ms suggests underlying sinus node dysfunction as the cause of symptoms attributed to bradycardia. It is of importance that other reasons for syncope, such as cerebral embolism or cerebral vascular insufficiency, are excluded by echocardiography and contrast angiography.

### *AV Block*

Intermittent AV block is diagnosed on the 24-hour ECG when the heart rate falls below 40 beats per minute with evidence of AV block. These patients should also undergo exercise testing because some of them may also suffer from chronotropic incompetence. Hence, the failure to increase heart rate with exercise testing or increased AV block may provide the criteria for insertion of a pacemaker. Furthermore, for patients with sinus node dysfunction, it is also important to assess AV node function. Usually, atrial pacing for determination of the Wenckebach point is all that is required. The Wenckebach point is that rate where nonconducted atrial beats are first produced. It should be >130 beats per minute. Not all electrophysiology laboratories routinely measure AV nodal (AH interval) or His-Purkinje (HV) conduction time intervals today.

## Selection of the Pacemaker

The selection of the type of pacemaker to be used will depend on whether nor not atrial fibrillation is present, on whether AV conduction is intact, and on the response of the sinus node to exercise on chronotropic competence testing.

In Table 3 are the types of permanent pacemaker units implanted in 408 patients during 1989 at our hospital. More than half (255) of the patients received a single chamber (VVI) pacemaker. The simplicity of implantation, low cost, and ease of positioning the electrode are the major reasons for our common use of VVI pacemakers.

Nevertheless, potential drawbacks to VVI pacemakers include loss of atrial transport function (especially important for patients with impaired diastolic function) and the pacemaker syndrome. The latter, which includes hypotension and eventually

**Table 3.** Types of pacemakers implanted at the University of Graz 1989

| | |
|---|---|
| VVI | 255 |
| DDD | 76 |
| VVI-R | 42 |
| DDD-R | 35 |
| Total | 408 |

congestive heart failure, is due to atrioventricular valve insufficiency caused by retrograde atrial stimulation in patients with retrograde (VA) conduction. Furthermore, up to 10% of patients with chronic VVI pacing will develop atrial fibrillation by 1 year, five times as many as with pacemakers that preserve atrial transport function [7] (DDD, AAI). Also, patients with VVI pacemakers are three times more liable to suffer stroke or heart failure than patients with DDD or AAI pacing [8].

It is our opinion that DDD pacing is to be preferred in patients with diastolic dysfunction due to coronary artery disease or cardiomyopathy. In these patients, optimal hemodynamics are provided by preserved atrial transport (DDD or AAI pacing) and the ability to increase rate as required. However, patients with atrial fibrillation must, of necessity, have a VVI pacemaker.

Those patients with heart block but without atrial fibrillation will only receive a VVI pacemaker if there is no retrograde conduction and if the bradyarrhythmias are infrequent [9]. A VVI-R pacemaker is prescribed in cases of ventricular chronotropic incompetence with atrial flutter or fibrillation. However, we note that rate-adaptive VVI pacemakers do not provide any hemodynamic advantage as long as the ejection fraction is within the normal range. If the ejection fraction is reduced, there is occasionally hemodynamic improvement when a VVI-R pacemaker is used. The explantation for hemodynamic improvement is that people with a reduced ejection fraction can optimize their ejection fraction only within a narrow range of paced rates. It should be tested beforehand whether or not the implantation of a VVI-R pacemaker in a patient with atrial flutter or fibrillation will lead to hemodynamic improvement [10]. In many cases, these patients do quite well with a VVI pacemaker.

Patients with the sick sinus syndrome rarely benefit from a VVI pacemaker because most have intact AV as well as VA conduction. VVI pacing with the latter could produce symptoms and complications of the pacemaker syndrome. Further, since AV conduction is intact, AAI pacing is preferred to preserve AV synchrony.

Patients with the carotid sinus syndrome only occasionally require pacing. In these cases, a ventricular demand (VVI) pacemaker programmed to a relatively low escape rate and with hysteresis function is most useful in our experience. By rate hysteresis is meant that the programmed escape interval is longer than the programmed automatic pacing interval to maximize the occurrence of spontaneous (sinus origin) rhythm. Alternatively stated, with rate hysteresis the time the pacemaker waits to initiate paced rhythm is longer than the time interval between paced beats once pacing has begun.

For patients with AV block, a VVI pacemaker is prescribed only if it provides adequate hemodynamic support and there is no retrograde (VA) conduction. In young patients, in whom a VVI pacemaker would not provide adequate hemodynamics, and who are not in atrial fibrillation, a DDD pacemaker is preferred by us. Further, if there is chronotropic incompetence, a DDD-R pacemaker is even more desirable. In patients with coronary heart disease, however, rate-adaptive pacing (DDD-R) can be less desirable because it can provoke ischemia.

Disadvantages of DDD pacemakers include the requirement for atrial and ventricular electrodes, a more complicated implantation procedure, the possibility of introducing atrial tachyarrhythmias (pacemaker-mediated tachycardia in patients with intact VA conduction), a higher complication rate and cost, and a more complicated patient follow-up procedure. The same, but only more so, applies to rate-adaptive DDD (DDD-R) pacemakers.

## Summary

A permanent pacemaker is indicated for any patient with sinus node dysfunction or AV block with symptoms attributable to bradycardia, and in whom hemodynamic improvement with relief of symptoms can be expected with pacing therapy. Before permanent pacing can be established, certain diagnostic testing may be required, including 24-hour (Holter) ECG monitoring, exercise testing, echocardiography, angiography, tilt testing, and pharmacological assessment of chronotropic competence. Invasive electrophysiological testing, including programmed atrial stimulation and His bundle recording, may be indicated in selected cases. Finally, the selection of the type of pacemaker to be used (VVI, VVI-R, AAI, AAI-R, DDD, DDD-R) will depend on such factors as underlying myocardial function, the nature of the patient's heart disease, the presence of intact AV or VA conduction, associated atrial fibrillation, the patient's age and life-style, and cost.

## References

1 Sutton R (1990) Cardiac pacing for bradyarrhythmias. Curr Opin Cardiol 5:74–79

2 Frye RL, Collins JJ, DeSanctis RW, Dodge HT, Dreifus LS, Fisch C, Gettes LS, Gillett PC, Parsonnet V, Reeves TJ, Weinberg SL (1984) Guidelines for permanent pacemaker implantation. May 1984, a report of the joint American College of Cardiology/American Heart Association task force on assessment of cardiovascular procedures. Circulation 70:331–339 A

3 Edhag O, Swhan S (1976) Prognosis of patients with complete heart block or arrhythmic syncope who were not treated with artificial pacemaker. Acta Med Scand 200:447–451

4 Dhingra RC, Denes P, Wu D, Wyndham CR, Amat-Y-Leon F, Towne W, Rosen KM (1976) Prospective observations in patients with chronic bundle branch block and marked H-V prolongation. Circulation 53:600–604

5 McAnulty JH, RAhimtoola SH, Murphy ES, Kauffman S, Ritzmann LW, Kanarek P, DeMots H (1978) A prospective study of sudden death in “high-risk” bundle-branch block. N Engl J Med 299:209–215

6 McAnulty JH, Rahimtoola SH, Murphy E, DeMots H, Ritzmann L, Kanarek PE, Kauffman S (1982) Natural history of “high-risk” bundle-branch block. N Engl J Med 307:137–143

7 Santini M, Alexidou G, Ansalone G, Cacciatore G, Cini R, Turitto G (1990) Relation of prognosis in sick sinus syndrome to age, conduction defects and modes of permanent pacing. Am J Cardiol 65:729–735

8 Sasaki S, Takeuchi A, Ohzeki M, Kishida H, Nishimoto T, Kakimoto S, Fukumoto H 81983) Long-term follow-up of paced patients with sick sinus syndrome. Pace 6:A–121
9 Morgan JM, Joseph SP, Bahri AK, Ramdial J, Crowther A (1990) Choosing the pacemaker; a rational approach to the use of modern pacemaker technology. Eur Heart J 11:753–764
10 Tyers FO (1990) Current status of sensor-modulated rate-adaptive cardiac pacing. J Am Coll Cardiol 15:412–418

# Place of Pacing in Cardiopulmonary Resuscitation

D. Dacar, K. H. Tscheliessnigg, F. Iberer and H. Gombotz

Symptomatic bradycardia of varying etiology may require electric stimulation of the heart even during the performance of other emergency procedures. Over the years, methods of pacemaker therapy that are suitable for application in emergency situations have been developed.

## Historical Background

In 1952, electrical stimulation of the heart was introduced into clinical practice by Zoll. It was first used as an external noninvasive method for the treatment of ventricular asystole or symptomatic bradycardia [1]. The application of subcutaneous needles combined with an extremely small stimulation area resulted in strong contraction of the underlying skeletal muscles and considerable burning pain during pacing at the electrode site. Also, the effectiveness of the stimulation could not be evaluated because of the stimulus-induced distortion of the surface ECG.

Another method of myocardial stimulation, applied mostly in emergencies, was introduced by Thevenet and colleagues in 1958 [2]. Based on the method described by Hyman in 1932 [3], a stimulation electrode was advanced over a trocar through the chest wall into the myocardium. As this is a potentially dangerous procedure (owing to possible injury to the heart and neighboring organs) and successful stimulation is the exception rather than the rule, this method has not been widely used.

In 1958 the transvenous method of cardiac stimulation was introduced by Furman and Robinson and soon proved superior to previously described methods [4]. At first, transvenous pacing was used only for temporary pacing, that is in emergency and standby situations.

Transesophageal electrodes were first used for cardiac defibrillation in 1956 by Whipple and Penton [5] and for cardioversion in 1966 by McNally and colleagues [6]. Subsequently (1968), Burack and Furman described transesophageal pacing as yet another indirect method for stimulation of the heart [7].

A modified system for noninvasive transcutaneous cardiac pacing was introduced in 1981 [8]. Large adhesive electrodes reduced muscle contractions and pain associated with transcutaneous pacing to a much more bearable extent.

## Suitability of Various Routes of Cardiac Pacing for Emergency Care

The first method, transcutaneous heart stimulation with subcutaneous electrodes [1], was soon abandoned because of serious side-effects, including local stimulation pain, muscle contraction, and inability to ascertain capture due to stimulus-induced distortion of the surface ECG.

Transthoracic stimulation described by Thevenet [2] produced even more serious complications. The associateed risks of producing intrathoracic complications or injury (hemopneumothorax, hemopericardium with cardiac tamponade, direct damage to the heart) and the uncertain ability to stimulate the heart were not conducive to widespread acceptance of the technique. Consequently, transthoracic pacing is rarely used today, and then only as a desperate measure in some cases.

For a long time transvenous stimulation was the preferred method for emergency pacing during resuscitation. This method is still uncontested for cases of standby-stimulation or as a temporary pacing method until a permanent pacemaker system can be implanted. However, application of transvenous pacing under emergency circumstances can have serious disadvantages. First, insertion and positioning of transvenous electrodes have to be performed under strictly sterile conditions. Second, experienced personnel and often x-ray equipment are also required. Pulmonary artery catheters adapted for pacing (Pacing TD, Paceport, AV Paceport, Baxter Healthcare, Santa Ana, CA, USA) can be inserted without x-ray. Third, implantation of transvenous pacing leads, even when performed by an experienced team, can take several minutes and often interferes with other necessary resuscitative procedures. Finally, since the transvenous method is invasive, there is the potential for serious complications (Table 1) [9, 10].

The transesophageal route is well suited for emergency pacing [7, 11–14]. Atrial as well as ventricular stimulation is possible in most cases. However, the conscious patient may not tolerate the insertion of the electrode. Some will experience moderate or severe burning with stimulation or discomfort due to diaphragmatic stimulation. For these reasons emergency transesophageal pacing is generally reserved for intubated or sedated patients.

Modified transcutaneous cardiac pacing [8] offers several advantages for emergency care. Sterile conditions are not required for external pacing. Transcutaneous pacing does not have to be performed by a specialized team, and the time required to obtain effective stimulation is on the average less than 1 min. Finally, institution of pacing does not interfere with other steps taken during basic resuscitation. To judge the effectiveness of transcutaneous stimulation, capture can be confirmed by appropriate filter-

**Table 1.** Complications of transvenous pacing

| | |
|---|---|
| Pneumothorax | Pulmonary embolism |
| Hemothorax | Sepsis |
| Ventricular perforation | Initiation of ventricular arrhythmia |
| Pericardial tamponade | Induction of complete heart block (with preexisting LBBB) |

LBBB, left bundle branch block

ing out of pacemaker stimulus artifacts during stimulation [15]. Transcutaneous pacing, however, also has some disadvantages. In varying percentages of patients (9%–60%) stimulation is ineffective [15–17, 21]. Even though large stimulation electrodes are used, some nonsedated patients will experience pain (21%–25%) [15, 21] or will not tolerate skeletal muscle stimulation with transcutaneous pacing (7%–8%) [15, 21].

## Evaluation of Emergency Pacing During Resuscitations

Surveys on the application of cardiac pacing under emergency circumstances have yielded varying results with regard to the outcome. The survival rate, especially when related to ultimate discharge from the hospital, is very low in some investigations [17–19]. In some reports [18, 20], no significant differences in survival have been found when patients with and without cardiac stimulation during resuscitation are compared. In contrast to these reports, however, there exist surveys with promising results with respect to survival in stimulated patients [15, 21, 22]. There are also case reports which describe significant hemodynmaic improvements with emergency pacing in cardiac patients [23, 24]. The reason for such divergent results lies partly in different pacing indications and noncomparable patient groups. Different survival rates also seem to have been dependent on the type of dysrhythmia which first presented during resuscitation. The best results were found in patients with supraventricular arrhythmias [15]; outcome was less favorable in patients with ventricular brady- or tachyarrhythmias [17]. Patients with asystole had the worst prognosis [17], possibly due to irreversible myocardial ischemia or massive infarction.

Temporary stimulation of the heart has become an indispensable procedure in cardiac emergencies today. Cardiac pacing should be applied as soon as possible, and not simply used as a last resort after ineffective drug therapy. The survival rate of patients requiring pacing therapy as part of cardiopulmonary resuscitation is as high as for those who do not require emergency pacing. It might be that improvement in survival would result from earlier institution of temporary pacing and improved means of accomplishing such pacing.

## Recommendations for Emergency Pacing

In the majority of cases, *transcutaneous stimulation* is the most practical available method. Its advantages are fast application and generally reliable stimulation effectiveness without restrictive side-effects or complications. *Transesophageal stimulation* nearly equals the transcutaneous method, although it is not widely available. The transesophageal pacing route may prove superior to transcutaneous pacing since it provides atrial stimulation, can be used for treatment of paroxysmal supraventricular tachycardia and atrial flutter, and will aid in electrophysiological diagnosis. Under emergency circumstances, the *transvenous method* should only be applied in the emergency room, operating room, or cath-lab under sterile conditions, and also with the availability of x-ray equipment and experienced personnel. Finally, *percutaneous transthoracic pacing* is considered obsolete today.

## References

1 Zoll PM (1952) Resuscitation of heart in ventricular standstill by external electrical stimulation. N Engl J Med 247:768–771
2 Thevenet A, Hodges PC, Lillehei CW (1958) Use of a myocardial electrode inserted percutaneously for control of complete atrioventricular block by an artificial pacemaker. Dis Chest 34:621–624
3 Hyman AS (1932) Resuscitation of the stopped heart by intracardial therapy. II. Experimental use of an artificial pacemaker. Arch Intern Med 50:283–286
4 Furman S, Robinson G (1958) Use of an intracardiac pacemaker in the correction of total heart block. Surg Forum 9:245–248
5 Whipple GH, Penton GB (1956) Transesophageal ventricular defibrillation. Clin Res Proc 4:105–108
6 McNally EM, Meyer EC, Langendorf R (1966) Elective countershock in unanesthetized patients with use of an esophageal electrode. Circulation 33:124–127
7 Burack B, Furman S (1969) Transesophageal cardiac pacing. Am J Cardiol 23:469–472
8 Zoll RH, Zoll PM, Belgard AH (1981) External noninvasive electric stimulation of the heart. Crit Care Med 9:393–397
9 Austin JL, Preis LK, Crampton RS, Beller GA, Martin RP (1982) Analysis of pacemaker malfunction and complications of temporary pacing in the coronary care unit. Am J Cardiol 49:301–306
10 Hynes JK, Holmes DR Jr, Harrison CE (1983) Five-year experience with temporary pacemaker therapy in the coronary care unit. Mayo Clin Proc 58:122–126
11 Gallagher JJ (1985) Esophageal pacing: diagnostic and therepeutic uses. In: Barold S (ed) Modern cardiac pacing, Futura, Mount Kisco, pp 783–798
12 Touborg P, Anderson HR, Pless P (1982) Low current bedside emergency atrial and ventricular cardiac pacing from the esophagus. Lancet i:166
13 Egorov DF, Sapozhnikov IR, Vygovskii AB, Domashenko AA, Zhukov OS (1987) Experience in using transesophageal electrocardiostimulation in emergency heart rhythm disorders. Ter Arkh 59:51–53
14 Lucet V, Do Ngoc D, Denjoy I, Saby MA, Toumieoux MC, Batisse A (1990) Esophageal pacing in children. 38 consecutive cases. Arch Fr Pediatr 47:185–189
15 Dunn DL, John JG (1989) Noninvasive temporary pacing: experience in a community hospital. Heart Lung 18:23–28
16 Heller MB, Peterson J, Ilkahpamipour K, Kaplan R, Paris PM (1989) A comparative study of five transcutaneous pacing devices in unanesthetized human volunteers. Prehosp Disaster Med 4:15–18
17 Rosenthal E, Thomas N, Quinn E, Chamberlain D, Vincent R (1988) Transcutaneous pacing for cardiac emergencies. PACE 11:2160–2167
18 Eitel DR, Guzzardi LJ, Stein SE, Drawbaugh RE, Hess DR, Walton SL (1987) Noninvasive transcutaneous cardiac pacing in prehospital cardiac arrest. Ann Emerg Med:531–534
19 Noe R, Cockrell W, Moses HW, Dove JT, Batchelder JE (1986) Transcutaneous pacemaker use in a large hospital. PACE 9:101–104
20 Hedges JR, Syverud SA, Dalsey WC, Feero S, Easter R, Shultz B (1987) Prehospital trial of emergency transcutaneous cardiac pacing. Circulation 76:1337–1343
21 Zoll PM, Zoll RH, Falk RH, Clinton JE, Eitel DR, Antman EM (1985) External noninvasive cardiac pacing: clinical trials. Circulation 71:937–944
22 Naumann d'Alnoncourt C, Becht I, v. Haase HJ, Helwing HP (1986) Nichtinvasive transkutane Stimulation des Herzens. Herzschrittmacher 6:5–9
23 Little T (1988) External cardiac pacing in right ventricular infarction. Ann Emerg Med 17:640–642
24 Cummins RO, Haulman J, Quan L, Graves JR, Peterson D, Horan S (1990) Near fatal yew berry intoxication treated with external cardiac pacing and digoxin specific FAB antibody fragments. Ann Emerg Med 19:38–43

# Holter Monitoring for Preoperative Assessment of Bradycardic Arrhythmias

H. METZLER, E. MAHLA, B. ROTMAN, H. GOMBOTZ, AND W.F. LIST

## Introduction

In many cases, severe bradycardic arrhythmias that produce unequivocal symptoms of hemodynamic insufficiency, and therefore are an indication for implantation of a temporary or permanent pacemaker before surgery, can be diagnosed with resting electrocardiography. Long-term (Holter) ECG monitoring may be required for less clear cases. The preoperative unit of our hospital occasionally uses 24-hour Holter ECG to identify patients at risk for or with bradycardic arrhythmias. The following study describes patients in whom the resting ECG and clinical symptoms led us to suspect severe bradycardic arrhythmias, and in whom 24–hour Holter ECG monitoring helped to confirm the diagnosis.

## Patients and Methods

All patients suspected of having symptomatic bradycardia and scheduled for elective, noncardiac surgery underwent routine preoperative assessment consisting of history, physical examination, resting (12 lead) ECG, chest x-ray, basic spirometry, and routine laboratory tests. Indications for preoperative 24-hour Holter ECG monitoring are

**Table 1.** Indications for preoperative 24-hour Holter ECG

1. Syncope, dizziness, or other symptoms possibly related to cardiac arrhythmias
2. Suspected paroxysms of supraventricular tachycardia, prolonged Q-T interval, R on T phenomenon
3. Rhythm disturbances in patients with significant cardiac disease such as cardiomyopathy, aortic stenosis, or mitral valve prolapse
4. Rhythm disturbances for which antiarrhythmic drug therapy has been prescribed
5. Recent myocardial infarction with arrhythmias and/or left ventricular dysfunction
6. Recent myocarditis with arrhythmias
7. Suspected sick sinus syndrome
8. Previous known or suspected intraoperative cardiac complication

listed in Table 1. Low serum potassium or magnesium levels, a digoxin level over 2 ng/ml, hyperthyroidism, congestive heart failure, or hypoxemia were ruled out before 24-hour Holter ECG monitoring. Patients in whom arrhythmias were most probably due to a cerebral tumor were also excluded.

Holter ECGs were obtained with ambulatory equipment (Tracker Reynolds, Hertfort, England) with a two-channel recorder. All Holter equipment and procedures were in accordance with specifications of the American Heart Association [1]. All patients were Holter monitored for 24 h. Monitor tapes were evaluated by a cardiologist immediately after the study period.

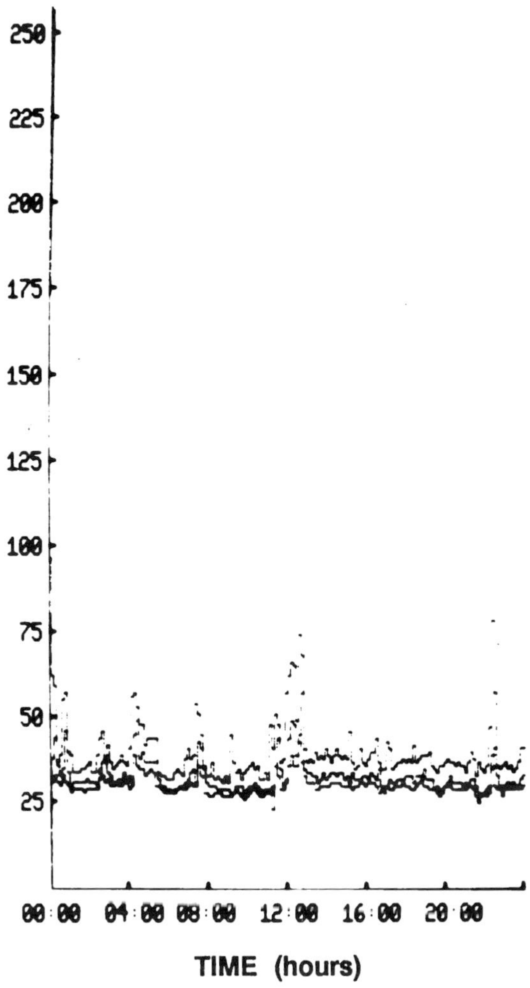


**Fig. 1.** Holter record from one patient with severe bradycardia and history of syncope. Average heart rate over 24 h was 34 beats/min. Minimum heart rate was 26 beats/min and maximum heart rate 97 beats/min

**Table 2.** Demographic and clinical data of patients selected for 24-hour Holter monitoring

| Patient | Age (Yrs) | Sex | Diagnosis | Holter Indication | Resting ECG | Holter Report | Therapy | Intraoperative Cardiovascular Problems |
|---|---|---|---|---|---|---|---|---|
| W.A. | 77 | m | Kidney tumor | Syncope | SR 42 bpm | Normal | – | – |
| S.A. | 80 | f | Urethral prolapse | Syncope | SA 56 bpm | SP up to 2000 ms<br>L IVb | P-PMI | – |
| N.H. | 59 | m | Cholecystitis | Syncope | SR 50 bpm | L IVb | Propafenone | – |
| L.C. | 77 | f | Hip surgery | History of intraoperative cardiac arrest | SR 67 bpm | L IVa | – | – |
| K.H. | 79 | f | Hip surgery | Syncope | SR 55 bpm | L IVa | – | – |
| L.M. | 78 | f | Inguinal hernia | Syncope | SR 50 bpm | SP up to 2400 ms<br>L IVa | P-PMI | – |
| B.I. | 72 | f | Carotid artery stenosis | Severe bradycardia during previous anesthesia | SR 70 bpm | L IVa | – | L IVb during induction of anesthesia |
| S.K. | 81 | m | Prostate hypertrophy | Syncope | SR 51 bpm | L IVb | Mexiletine | |
| K.J. | 70 | f | Colon tumor | Syncope | AF 95 bpm | L IVb | Propafenone | |

P–PMI, permanent pacemaker insertion; SR, sinus rhythm; SA, sinus arrhythmia; AF, atrial fibrillation; L, arrhythmias based on Lown classification (IVa or IVb — see text); SP, sinus pause

## Results

A total of 13,806 patients were seen at the preoperative unit between July 1987 and January 1990. Fifty-seven (0.4%) patients had indications for 24-hour Holter ECG monitoring (Table 1). Nine of these 57 patients (mean age 74 years) had a history of syncopal attacks or the presence of a potentially symptomatic bradycardic arrhythmia in the resting ECG. Table 2 provides further information regarding these patients. A severe bradycardic disorder was confirmed in two patients who showed a sinus rhythm with sinus pauses of 2000 to 2400 ms while awake as well as Lown class IVa or IVb arrhythmia. The former are couplets of ventricular ectopic beats and the latter runs of ventricular ectopic beats (triplets and more). Both patients underwent implantation of a permanent pacemaker with local anesthesia before surgery. Three patients with Lown IVb arrhythmias received antiarrhythmic treatment with propafenone or mexiletine. One patient with Lown IVa arrhythmias and sinus bradycardia of 45 bpm developed Lown IVb arrhythmias during induction of anesthesia. All other patients were free of intraoperative and postoperative cardiac complications. Figure 1 illustrates the 24-hour report of one patient with severe bradycardic episodes and a history of syncope.

## Discussion

The indications for temporary perioperative pacing or permanent implantation of a cardiac pacemaker are relatively straightforward [2–5]. Most bradycardic arrhythmias requiring a pacemaker can be identified by a resting ECG and the patient's history. Twenty-four hour Holter ECG monitoring is indicated only when symptoms and resting ECG findings fail to reveal a diagnosis. Our experience with 24-hour Holter ECG monitoring in patients scheduled for surgery has been reported previously [6]. The list of indications for the preoperative evaluation of arrhythmias (Table 1) does not differ significantly from that recently formulated in the United States [7].

Only 0.4% of the patients in our preoperative unit showed an indication for Holter monitoring. Most of these patients did not have bradycardic arrhythmias. However, 24-hour Holter ECG monitoring can provide a certain diagnosis in selected patients. It can differentiate between cardiac and noncardiac syncope, and establish whether cardiac syncope is due to tachycardic or to bradycardic arrhythmias. More precise diagnosis of cardiac syncope could be the basis for permanent pacemaker implantation, temporary perioperative pacing, or antiarrhythmic medication.

Most Holter ECGs are performed over a 24-hour period. This duration of monitoring is now widely used because (1) it can register most, if not all, ECG phenomena subject to a circadian rhythm, and (2) there is also a high probability of documenting events that trigger an actual syncopal attack [3, 7, 8]. However, longer periods of Holter monitoring may occasionally be required to evaluate syncope. An underlying, bradycardic disorder of cardiac impulse formation and/or conduction occurs less often than ventricular extrasystoles. For the latter, monitoring for more than 24 h is not expected to greatly improve the detection rate of 85% [9]. In contrast, evidence of abnormal sinus node function has been reported to be identified in only about 25% of patients during the first 24 h of Holter monitoring [10]. Thus, longer Holter recording periods may be required to diagnose sinus node dysfunction as the cause of syncope. On the other hand, preoperative Holter testing should not unduly postpone scheduled surgery.

Holter cardiac monitoring confirmed the presence of bradycardia or high grade ventricular arrhythmias in eight of the nine patients in the present series. This indicates appropriate use of 24-hour Holter for preoperative assessment of bradycardic arrhythmias in our preoperative unit. In our experience, less experienced personnel may be tempted to order Holter monitoring more often than indicated. This is contrary to a principal purpose of a preoperative unit, i.e., expediting preoperative evaluation of patients.

Bradycardic arrhythmias occur mainly in older patients. The mean age of the patients in this series was 74 years. Since increasing numbers of older patients are undergoing surgery, these patients may especially benefit from more extensive preoperative work-up. Furthermore, indicated treatment that might be instituted as the result of more thorough preoperative evaluation, including implantation of a pacemaker, will benefit the patient not only during the perioperative period but also following discharge from the hospital.

## References

1. Sheffield LT and the Task Force of the Committee on Electrocardiography and Cardiac Electrophysiology of the Council on Clinical Cardiography (1985) Recommendations for standards of instrumentation and practice in the use of ambulatory electrocardiography. Circulation 71: 626A–636A
2. Arbeitsgruppe Herzschrittmacher der Deutschen Gesellschaft für Herz- und Kreislaufforschung (1990) Empfehlungen zur Herzschrittmachertherapie. Herzschrittmacher Elektrophys 1: 42–51
3. Atlee JL (1990) Perioperative cardiac dysrhythmias, 2nd edn. Year Book, Chicago, pp 318–328
4. Stull MW, Luck JC, Martin DE (1990) Anesthesia for patients with electrophysiologic disorders. In: Hensley FA, Martin DE (eds) The practice of cardiac anesthesia. Little, Brown, Boston, pp 493–524
5. Frye RL, Collins JJ, De Sanctis RW, Dodge HT, Dreifus LS, Fisch C, Gettes LS, Gillett PC, Parsonnet V, Reeves TJ, Weinberg SL (1984) Guidelines for permanent cardiac pacemaker implantation, May 1984. A report of the joint American College of Cardiology/American Heart Associations task force on assessment of cardiovascular procedures. Circulation 70: 331A–339A
6. Metzler H, Rehak P, Mahla E, Rotman B, List WF (1990) Präoperative Risikoerfassung: Langzeitelektrokardiographie zur gezielten Arrhythmiediagnostik. Anaesthesist 39: 77–82
7. Knoebel SB, Crawford MH, Dunn MI, Fisch C, Forrester JS, Hutter AM, Kennedy HL, Lux RL, Sheffield LT (1989) Guidelines for ambulatory electrocardiography. Circulation 79: 206–215
8. Kennedy HL, Chandra V, Sayter KL, Caranis DG (1978) Effectiveness of increasing hours of continuous ambulatory electrocardiography in detecting maximal ventricular ectopy. Am J Cardiol 42:925
9. Schmidt G, Goedel-Meinen L, Wirtzfeld A (1986) Diagnostik von Herzrhythmusstörungen. Tempo Medical, Munich, pp 24–25
10. Lekieffre J, Libersa C, Caron J, Pladys A, Carre A (1984) Electrocardiographic aspects of sinus node dysfunction: use of the Holter electrocardiographic recording. In: Levy S, Schinman MM (eds) Cardiac arrhythmias: from diagnosis to therapy. Futura, Mount Kisco, p 74

# Temporary Perioperative Pacing

J.L. ATLEE

## Introduction

Temporary pacing has distinct advantages over drugs for the management of most cases of bradycardia and many tachyarrhythmias that occur in perioperative settings. The chief advantage is that pacing will remove or reduce the requirement for chronotropic or antiarrhythmic drugs, which drugs may be ineffective, worsen arrhythmias, or cause other circulatory imbalance. Additionally, pacing can be instituted or terminated at will, in direct contrast to drugs. A limitation to more pervasive use of temporary pacing, however, has been the lack of effective noninvasive methods. Nevertheless, emerging interest in the relatively noninvasive transcutaneous and transesophageal pacing routes may ultimately remove existing barriers to more extensive use of temporary pacing in the perioperative environment.

Discussed in this chapter are methods and indications for temporary pacing, as well as the application of temporary pacing to the management of specific cardiac rhythm disturbances.

## Methods for Temporary Pacing

How aggressive anesthesiologists or critical care specialists are with applying temporary pacing methods for arrhythmia management depends on the types of patients encountered and his or her familiarity and confidence with available temporary pacing equipment. As already noted, a real limitation to the more widespread use of temporary pacing has been the lack of suitable noninvasive methods. *Transvenous (endocardial) electrodes* are too invasive for most prophylactic use. Further, optimal electrode positioning often requires fluoroscopy or x-rays, particularly with atrial or atrioventricular (AV) sequential pacing leads, and can be difficult or time-consuming under emergency circumstances. *Pacing versions of pulmonary artery catheters (PAC)* can also be used to provide endocardial pacing (Pacing TD, Paceport, A-V Paceport, Baxter Healthcare, Irvine, CA). Advantages of pacing PAC over other transvenous pacing leads include no requirement for fluoroscopy or x-ray for positioning (usually), and PAC insertion is a familiar procedure for most anesthesiologists. Nevertheless, pacing PAC must be considered invasive, and they are too expensive for routine use. Temporary transvenous pacing as a prophylactic measure is most likely to be used in patients undergoing open heart surgery. However, transvenous pacing is generally used only during the prebypass period, since *epicardial pacing wires* are more or less routinely placed post-bypass by most cardiac surgeons.

*Transcutaneous, indirect ventricular pacing* has been suggested for emergency pacing of bradycardia and asystole [1], although there are potential limitations to this technique. Included are the inability to obtain capture in all patients (e.g., those which morbid obesity, pericardial effusion, pulmonary emphysema) and the failure of transcutaneous ventricular pacing to preserve atrial transport function. Since diastolic ventricular filling is both active (result of atrial contraction) and passive (result of flow created by pressure gradients between the atria and ventricles), atrial transport function can be critical in patients with failing or noncompliant (stiff) ventricles and high filling pressures. Such impaired ventricular diastolic function might be produced by myocardial disease (e.g., coronary insufficiency, hypertensive cardiomyopathy), the effects of aging itself, or even by inhalation anesthetics [2–8].

These limitations of transcutaneous pacing are not ones expected with *transesophageal indirect atrial pacing (TAP)*. However, TAP does require intact AV conduction, and at least most atrial beats should be conducted to the ventricles at physiologic atrial rates. Further, TAP is not effective in patients with chronic atrial fibrillation. Theoretically, in patients with bradycardia due to sinus node dysfunction and attacks of paroxysmal (acute) atrial fibrillation, direct current cardioversion could be used to terminate atrial fibrillation. TAP could then be used for bradycardia following conversion and prevention of recurrences. Antitachycardia pacing with TAP electrodes is also effective treatment for atrial flutter (type 1) and paroxysmal (reentrant) supraventricular tachycardia [9–14].

TAP systems employing a pill electrode have recently been marketed in the USA and elsewhere (Arzco Medical Systems, Vernon Hills, IL). These are used for noninvasive electrophysiologic testing and stress pacing in conscious patients. Pill electrodes, however, are not suitable for emergency pacing in unconcious or anesthetized patients for obvious reasons. We are presently working to adapt TAP for use with disposable esophageal stethoscopes in unconcious or anesthetized patients, and have shown the feasibility (reliable atrial capture with low pacing thresholds) of this approach in anesthetized surgical patients [15]. In this same study of 100 patients, an approximate 40% incidence of sinus bradycardia or AV junctional rhythms was found. TAP at about 80 beats/min produced substantial and statistically significant hemodynamic improvement. A subsequent case report describes the use of TAP to provide hemodynamic support in two patients with severe bradycardia that did not respond to chronotropic drug therapy [16]. At present, we are performing clinical testing of disposable esophageal stethoscopes with atrial pacing electrodes. In addition to determining TAP thresholds, we are also documenting any use of TAP for treatment of brady(tachy)cardic arrhythmias, as well as hemodynamic effects of TAP when used to treat arrhythmias. Another study will determine optimum paced rates (TAP) for patients with cardiovascular disease. Further, we are testing designs of disposable esophageal stethoscopes with additional electrodes for ventricular pacing and recording, including signal-averaged and high-frequency-processed ECG for more specific and sensitive diagnosis, and earlier detection, of myocardial ischemia. Finally, we will test these electrodes alone or with surface or other intracavitary electrodes to perform direct current cardioversion and defibrillation. We expect lower current requirements than possible with surface electrodes alone.

## Indications for Temporary Pacing

### *Pacing for Bradycardia*

The new occurrence of hemodynamically significant bradycardia due to advanced second-degree AV block or complete third-degree AV block is uncommon in patients undergoing anesthesia and surgery in the absence of acute myocardial infarction, unless the patient sustains direct injury to the conducting system due to surgical, electrical, or mechanical causes, including manipulation of intravascular catheters. However, hemodynamically deleterious bradycardia due to sinus node dysfunction (consequent to disease, physiologic imbalance, or drugs), AV junctional rhythm disturbances, or excessive vagal tone (e.g., oculocardiac reflex) is not uncommon during anesthesia and surgery.

At least a tendency toward bradycardia is expected with narcotic-based anesthetic techniques, especially when muscle relaxants that are devoid of autonomic side effects or do not cause histamine release are used. Further, if drugs with central $\alpha_2$-adrenergic agonist activity (e.g., clonidine, dexmedetomidine) come into general use as prophylactic measures against hypertension, tachycardia, or arrhythmias provoked by airway or surgical manipulation, the incidence of hemodynamically disadvantageous bradycardia could become even higher.

While modest bradycardia could be advantageous in patients with ischemic heart disease, and is relatively innocuous in the absence of any heart disease, severe sinus bradycardia ($\leq$ 50 beats/min) will likely cause at least some circulatory insufficiency in all anesthetized patients. Bradycardic AV junctional or ventricular escape rhythms with loss of atrial transport function (also atrial fibrillation with too slow ventricular rates) will likely produce at least some circulatory insufficiency in all patients. The same rhythms in patients with impaired ventricular diastolic function due to advanced age or ischemic, hypertensive, or dilated cardiomyopathy can be hemodynamically ineffective and lead to cardiovascular collapse if not treated promptly.

Based on the above, it is apparent that bradycardic arrhythmias will be tolerated by some but not all patients. Tolerance will depend most on underlying myocardial function (those with diastolic dysfunction might be most affected) and less on the actual rate of the disturbance, although increased rate and contractility are the only mechanisms available to increase cardiac output in the patient with chronic atrial fibrillation. Consequently, I believe that the anesthesiologist should no longer view bradyarrhythmias as benign disturbances in all patients. Unfortunately, data are lacking at this time to substantiate this claim for perioperative circumstances, although there is ample hemodynamic data to substantiate this claim for patients who have had permanent pacemaker systems implanted for symptomatic bradycardia. Perhaps a major reason why many anesthesiologists view bradycardia as relatively benign is that they lack effective treatment for most cases. Chronotropic drugs are often not the solution because they can produce untoward tachycardia, are ineffective, or produce far worse rhythm disturbances [16].

Concerning *pacing methods to be used for treating bradycardia,* because an investigational TAP system is available to us and TAP is noninvasive, we are quite aggressive in using transesophageal pacing in any patient scheduled for anesthesia and surgery believed prone to circulatory insufficiency from bradycardic arrhythmias. Likely candidates include patients with hypertension or coronary artery disease who are receiving calcium channel or β-adrenergic blockers, as well as patients with proven or suspected sinus node dysfunction who are undergoing cardiothoracic, major vascular, or other complicated or extensive surgical procedures. TAP might also be used in patients with proven or suspected bradycardia-dependent tachyarrhythmias (e.g., long QT interval). These same indications will likely be at least the initial ones for TAP as disposable esophageal stethoscopes designed for TAP become commercially available over the next several years. Until TAP is available for clinical use, and especially if pulmonary artery pressure monitoring is planned, one should consider pacing versions of PAC for any of the forementioned pacing indications. The decision to insert a pacing pulmonary catheter that can provide atrial or AV sequential pacing will depend on whether or not the patient has intact AV conduction or chronic atrial fibrillation, and clinical estimates (or actual measurements) of diastolic ventricular function. Finally, a transcutaneous pacing system should at least be available to all operating rooms and postanesthesia or intensive care units.

A firm indication for temporary transvenous (endocardial) pacing in perioperative settings is any patient with clearly documented symptoms or signs of circulatory insufficiency due to bradycardia, whatever the cause. In these patients, the transvenous pacing capability should be established prior to operation. The cardiac chamber(s) to be paced will depend on the nature and cause of bradycardia, accompanying rhythm disturbances, and available pacing equipment.

Uncertainty exists concerning the need for temporary pacing in patients with *bifascicular heart block.* Bifascicular block is block of any two of the three major divisions of the common (His) bundle, i.e., the right bundle branch and anterior or posterior fascicles of the left bundle branch. However, there is no available evidence that such block, in the absence of acute or evolving myocardial infarction, will progress to complete heart block with anesthesia and surgery. Therefore, prophylactic transvenous pacing is not indicated for all patients with bifascicular heart block. Bifascicular block with symptoms clearly attributable to bradycardia is, however, a firm indication for temporary transvenous pacing in perioperative settings.

Also, concerning indications for perioperative transvenous pacing of patients with bradycardia, it may be that bradycardia does not produce symptoms or signs of circulatory insufficiency. Bradycardia in these patients is, however, associated with unstable escape rhythms. Since anesthetics and drugs used to suppress escape rhythms are likely to worsen bradycardia, prophylactic temporary pacing for these patients should be given careful consideration.

Finally, it is now appreciated by almost all cardiovascular surgeons that brady (tachy)cardic rhythm disturbances are quite common in cardiac surgical patients following cardiopulmonary bypass. Therefore, most centers today more or less routinely insert temporary epicardial pacing wires as a prophylactic measure in these patients.

*Pacing for tachyarrhythmias*

Temporary pacing can be effective treatment for many tachyarrhythmias, particularly those of supraventricular origin and due to reentry of excitation. In fact, temporary pacing is the preferred method following open heart surgery, if temporary pacing wires are in place. Advantages and disadvantages of antitachycardia pacing are listed in Table 1, and pacing modes used against tachyarrhythmias listed in Table 2. Not every mode of pacing for tachycardia can be accomplished by all available models of temporary pulse generators, and some are more effective than others for terminating specific tachyarrhythmias. Regardless, any form of antitachycardia pacing should be undertaken only with direct current (DC) cardioversion and defibrillation available as a backup measure. This is because pacing could fail to terminate the tachyarrhythmia and cardioversion would then be indicated, or pacing might initiate potentially lethal tachyarrhythmias, including ventricular fibrillation. Also, with DC cardioversion as compared to pacing therapy, the distinction between supraventricular and ventricular mechanisms for the rhythm disturbance is not so important.

**Table 1.** Advantages and disadvantages of temporary antitachycardia pacing

| Advantages | Disadvantages |
|---|---|
| Treat tachyarrhythmias promptly without drugs | Inability to terminate some tachyarrhythmias |
| No need to titrate drugs or other measures to effect | May accelerate tachycardia or initiate new tachyarrhythmia |
| Avoid adverse effects of antiarrhythmic drugs | Some pacing modes require sophisticated pulse generators |
| Availability of pacing for any bradycardia or asystole posttermination | Present lack of suitable noninvasive equipment for routine perioperative use |

**Table 2.** Pacing modes used to terminate or suppress tachyarrhythmias

| Mode | Description |
|---|---|
| Underdrive pacing | Asynchronous pacing at a rate less than the tachycardia rate |
| Burst pacing | Asynchronous pacing (3 – 100 pulses or more) at a rate well in excess of tachycardia rate |
| Overdrive pacing | Asynchronous pacing (15 – 30 s or more) at rate 10%–15% above tachycardia rate |
| Programmed extrastimulation | Single, paired, or triple extrastimuli |

## Management of Specific Arrhythmias

### *Sinus Node Dysfunction*

Manifestations of sinus node dysfunction, commonly termed the sick sinus syndrome, consist of (1) persistent, severe, and unexpected sinus bradycardia; (2) brief or sustained sinus arrest with an escape rhythm, often of AV junctional origin; (3) prolonged sinus arrest with failure of all subsidiary pacemakers, resulting in cardiac asystole; (4) chronic atrial fibrillation with an unusually slow ventricular response not caused by drug therapy; (5) inability of the heart to resume normal sinus rhythm following direct current cardioversion for atrial fibrillation or flutter; and (6) alternating bradyarrhythmias with tachyarrhythmias [17].

Sinus node dysfunction may be due either to failure of impulse formation (automaticity) within the sinus node or to exit block from the sinus node to the perinodal atrial tissue as the result of conduction abnormalities [17]. Conduction delay from the sinus node to the perinodal cells can also lead to sinus node reentry and tachycardia in some instances. Since the AV node is rarely involved, the onset of atrial flutter or fibrillation in patients with sinus node dysfunction may lead to alternating bradycardic and tachycardic arrhythmias. Finally, the same supraventricular tachyarrhythmias that suppress sinus node automaticity through the mechanism of overdrive suppression may result in long periods of sinus arrest following termination of tachyarrhythmias, also a characteristic feature of the bradycardia-tachycardia syndrome.

While the foregoing describes in a general fashion manifestations of and mechanisms for intrinsic sinus node dysfunction, extrinsic factors unique to the perioperative environment are likely to contribute to or influence manifestations of sinus node dysfunction in affected patients. Included could be potentially adverse cardiac electrophysiologic effects of anesthetic and related drugs (largely unknown), autonomic or physiologic imbalance (also unknown), and interactions involving any of these. Therefore, it should not bc surprising that drugs commonly used to treat manifestations of sinus node dysfunction in patients with sinus node disease can at times be ineffective, aggravate sinus node dysfunction, or be the cause for more worrisome tachyarrhythmias or escape rhythms [16].

Consequently, while it has been cutomary to treat bradycardia, escape rhythms, and tachyarrhythmias resulting from sinus node dysfunction with chronotropic or antiarrhythmic drugs, this may not be the best practice. Electrical therapy, especially antibradycardia pacing as definitive or preventive (i.e., escape rhythms or bradycardia-dependent tachycardia) treatment, appears better. But, as already noted, limiting the more widespread application of pacing is the current unavailability of effective noninvasive methods. Since AV conduction is intact in most patients with sinus node dysfunction, and many are not in chronic atrial fibrillation (presumably at least not in the early stages of dysfunction), transesopageal atrial pacing (TAP) should be well-suited as definitive or preventive treatment for most patients with sinus node dysfunction [15, 16]. External pulse generators for TAP are commercially available (Arzco Medical Systems, Vernon Hills, IL). These can be used with standard transvenous pacing leads positioned in the esophagus, and disposable esophageal stethoscopes with TAP electrodes should be available (Arzco) within a year or two of publication of this book. IF TAP is not practical (e.g., esophageal disease) or available (standard external pulse generators generally provide insufficient current, except for infants or small children), then invasive temporary pacing methods are still preferred to drugs for most patients with serious manifestations of sinus node dysfunction. Atrial or AV sequential pacing (with AV conduction block) are the preferred pacing modes, since most patients with sinus node dysfunction have at least some impairment of ventricular diastolic function and will benefit from preserved atrial transport function (discussed above). For the same reason, transcutaneous indirect ventricular pacing should be used only as a temporary, life-saving measure for treatment of severe bradycardic escape rhythms. Additionally, if paroxysmal atrial tachyarrhythmias interfere with pacing, DC cardioversion or pacing methods (as indicated or applicable, discussed below) should be considered. Possibly drugs could be added for suppression or prevention of recurrences. Finally, sinus tachycardia, often a compensatory rhythm disturbance (or due to pain or inadequate anesthesia), is not amenable to pacing therapy or cardioversion. However, paroxysmal atrial tachycardia due to sinus node reentry (-PAT-SR) is not uncommon in patients with sinus node dysfunction and not easily distinguished from sinus tachycardia in acute circumstances. PAT-SR can be treated by pacing or cardioversion. Clues that to me suggest the diagnosis of PAT-SR as compared to sinus tachycardia in clinical settings include: (1) much *faster rate* (≥ 150–160 beats/min) than can ordinarily be achieved by the sinus node in most patients with sinus node dysfunction; (2) *abrupt onset,* often following a premature beat, versus a more gradual acceleration in rate; (3) *abrupt termination* (if spontaneous), followed by sinus pause or arrest; and (4) *appearance* of P waves, which are similar to those of sinus-origin beats.

### *Ectopic Atrial Beats or Tachycardia*

The adjective "ectopic" is used to distinguish the presumed electrophysiologic mechanim(s) for these rhythm disturbances, which could be automaticity (normal or abnormal) or triggerered activity or automaticity [18]. Since these rhythm disturbances are due to an automatic or triggered as opposed to a reentrant mechanism, they are not easily interrupted or terminated by pacing. Atrial ectopic beats may be suppressed by pacing, however, but this is usually done only if such beats initiate paroxysms of supraventricular tachycardia. Ectopic atrial tachycardia (EAT) is most often faster than 140 beats/min, with 2:1 or variable AV block present. AV block is not a feature of paroxysmal (reentrant) forms of supaventricular tachycardia. Due to AV block and resulting ventricular rate reduction, it may not be necessary to provide any form of therapy for EAT. Without AV block, drugs (digitalis, β- or calcium channel blockers) can be used to slow AV conduction, and overdrive atrial pacing at a rate in excess of that of EAT may be used as an alternative means to drugs for slowing AV conduction [11]. With the latter, the atrial paced rate is set fast enough to produce 2:1 AV block. If all these measures fail to provide sufficient ventricular rate reduction, burst pacing at a rate 10%–15% faster than the EAT rat for 30 s will occasionally interrupt EAT or will initiate atrial fibrillation [11]. Atrial fibrillation could be preferred to EAT because ventricular rate reduction is easier with the former. Finally, due to the risk of triggering ventricular fibrillation, cardioversion is not recommended if EAT is or could be due to digitalis.

*AV Junctional Rhythm (AVJR) and Tachycardia (AVJT)*

These two rhythm disturbances are distinguished solely by rate criteria (AVJR ≤ 80 beats/min). AVJR is common in healthy young adults, especially with any of the potent volatile anesthetics. In this case, it often presents as isorhythmic AV dissociation. With the latter, the atrial and AV junctional rates are nearly matched, so that P waves appear to march in and out of the QRS complex. AVJR and AVJT are common in patients with ischemic heart disease and following open heart surgery. AVJT is rarely faster than 120–130 beats/min in adult patients. Either AVJR or AVJT can be extremely disadvantageous to patients with impaired myocardial function, and especially with diastolic ventricular dysfunction. Both AVJR and AVJT are easily suppressed by atrial or AV sequential pacing at a rate just above that of the rhythm disturbance. TAP is quite effective for this purpose. Once capture is obtained, the initial paced rate is maintained for a period (variable) and then gradually reduced over a period of minutes to hours as sinus rhythm is restored. Occasionally, AVJT can be so fast as to be life-threatening (most often in infants following open heart surgery). In such cases, ventricular paired pacing may be attempted to improve hemodynamics [11]. Paired pacing, which requires a temporary pulse generator that can provide extra stimuli (e.g., model 5326 programmable stimulator, Medtronic, Minneapolis, MN), is performed as follows. Ventricular pacing is carried out at some predetermined rate, but with a stimulated premature beat following every paced beat. Paired pacing doubles the ventricular electrical rate, but the effective contractile rate is halved.

*Paroxysmal (Reentrant) Supraventricular Tachycardia (PSVT)*

Most sudden-onset (hence, paroxysmal) SVT is initiated by a premature atrial beat, or sometimes AV junctional or ventricular beats if retrogradely conducted to the atria. The site of reentry that sustains PSVT is commonly (40%–50%) the AV node, with fast and slow pathway dissociation. Perhaps equally or somewhat less common is a reentry loop involving the AV node and an accessory (AV bypass) pathway. The bypass pathway may manifest itself in some patients with ventricular preexcitation (e.g., Wolff-Parkinson-White syndrome) or may be concealed (sustains only retrograde VA conduction). Less common reentry sites for PSVT are the sinus node (10%–15%) and atria (< 5%). The reentry site is often difficult to establish without electrophysiologic study, and should matter little for acute management. Atrial underdrive or overdrive pacing can be used to interrupt PSVT [11]. With atrial underdrive pacing (pacing can also be performed from ventricles in patients with functional VA conduction), it is possible that one or more properly timed beats during pacing (a chance occurrence) will interrupt the reentry loop. Underdrive pacing is performed at a rate slower than that of the tachycardia. Overdrive pacing, the other method, is performed at a rate faster (10%–15%) than that of the tachycardia. Once atrial capture is evident, the overdrive rate is sustained for 30 s, then abruptly or gradually slowed to some predetermined rate. If the mechanism for PSVT involves retrograde conduction through an AV bypass pathway, then overdrive pacing must be performed at a rate considerably faster than that of PSVT in order to produce bidirectional conduction block in the reentry loop. Finally, recurrences of PSVT might be prevented by atrial asynchronous pacing in an attempt to suppress premature beats initiating PSVT.

*Atrial Fibrillation*

Atrial fibrillation cannot be terminated by pacing, but is with DC cardioversion. However, if the ventricular rate with atrial fibrillation is too slow, ventricular pacing should be considered to provide rate support.

*Atrial Flutter*

Type II atrial flutter (atrial rate >340 beats/min) is not responsive to pacing, but is to DC cardioversion. Type I atrial flutter (atrial rate <340 beats/min) is treated by atrial overdrive pacing in a manner similar to that for PSVT. At least with direct atrial pacing, it is preferable to perform pacing with electrodes positioned on or in the high right atrium to increase the likelihood of recognizing atrial capture during pacing [11]. Atrial flutter waves are typically negative or biphasic in the inferior leads, but positive with capture when pacing from high in the atrium. With (indirect) TAP, the large pacing artifacts may make it next to impossible to diagnose capture from P wave appearance alone. Regardless, once atrial capture is suspected or evident, pacing is continued for at least 30 s, then gradually or abruptly slowed. Gradual slowing is preferred in patients with sinus node dysfunction in order to reduce the likelihood of bradycardia or asystole following termination of atrial flutter. In addition to duration of pacing (≥ 30 s), the current strength should be high (20 mA) with transvenous or epicardial leads, and at least twice threshold with TAP. Finally, while sinus rhythm is often restored using these methods, transient or even persistent atrial fibrillation are not uncommon following cessation of pacing. Neverthelees, ventricular rate reduction is much easier with atrial fibrillation than with flutter.

*Idioventricular Rhythm (IVR) and Ventricular Tachycardia (VT)*

IVR has similar causes to AV junctional rhythm (except that it is not caused by potent inhalation anesthetics), and is treated with atrial or AV sequential overdrive pacing, depending on whether or not AV conduction is intact. Slow monomorphic VT (≤ 120 beats/min), also termed idioventricular tachycardia, has the same causes and treatment (overdrive pacing) as AVJT.

Several modes of pacing have been used more or less successfully with other forms of VT [11]. Included are ventricular extrastimulation and ventricular overdrive and paired and burst pacing. Any of these methods should be attempted only with a DC cardiovertor/defibrillator present, and probably only by persons quite familiar with cardiac electrophysiologic methods. Also, with immediate danger of cardiovascular collapse, no time should be wasted attempting any pacing method. With extrastimulation, single, paired, or triple extra stimuli may be effective, but the site of stimulation may be the most important factor. The same is true for ventricular overdrive pacing, but it is also necessary to pace at a rate considerably faster than the VT rate. Ventricular paired pacing is performed the same way and for similar reasons as mentioned earlier for AVJT. Finally, burst pacing of the ventricles is carried out for 5–7 capture beats at a rate 40–50 beats/min above the VT rate. If this fails, pacing is next carried out for 10–12 beats at the same rate. This sequence is repeated with 25 beat/min increases in paced rate, or DC cardioversion is used. Once VT is terminated by any of the above pacing methods or cardioversion, and the atrial or ventricular rate is too slow, atrial, AV sequential, or ventricular pacing may be used to suppress premature beats initiating recurrences of VT. Antibradycardia pacing is also used as prophylactic treatment for torsades de pointes VT, since it frequently occurs in association with bradycardic states.

### *Ventricular Fibrillation (VF)*

VF cannot be terminated by any form of pacing therapy. Neither is DC cardioversion effective, since R or S waves cannot be distinguished from T waves for proper discharge synchronization. Thus, DC defibrillation is the only effective treatment for VF, although pacing methods may be useful for treating some rhythm disturbances that occur before or after VF.

### *AV and Fascicular Heart Block*

As noted earlier, except with acute myocardial infarction or direct damage to the conducting system, bifascicular conduction block with in or below the common (His) bundle is not expected to progress to complete heart block during anesthesia and surgery. Thus, unless there are associated symptoms or signs clearly attributable to bradycardia, invasive temporary perioperative pacing is not indicated, although one may wish to establish central venous access for emergency transvenous pacing in some patients. The same dictum (significant associated bradycardia) also applies to first- and second-degree AV block. Type II (Mobitz) or advanced (two or more non-conducted atrial beats in sucession) second AV block and 3° (complete) AV block are usually symptomatic or produce some circulatory insufficiency, and therefore are indications for temporary perioperative pacing. Most patients with symptomatic bradycardia, however, will already have a permanent pacemaker. Pacing is always the preferred method for perioperative management of patients with symptomatic or hemodynamically deleterious bradycardia due to heart block, since drugs cannot be relied upon to safely or effectively increase the rate of lower pacemakers. Finally, the site chosen for temporary pacing (AV sequential vs ventricular) will largely depend on the duration and nature of the planned surgery, as well as the underlying myocardial functional state. In this regard, as already noted, patients with ventricular diastolic dysfunction are expected to benefit most from AV sequential pacing.

## References

1 Kelly JS, Royster RL (1989) Noninvasive transcutaneous cardiac pacing. Anesth Analg 69:229–238
2 Greenberg B, Chatterjee K, Parmley WW, Werner JA, Holly AN (1979) The influence of left atrial filling pressure on atrial contribution to cardiac output. Am Heart J 98: 742–751
3 Pearson AC, Janosik DL; Redd RM, Buckinham TA, Labovitz AJ (1989) Hemodynamic benefit of atrioventricular synchrony: prediction from baseline Doppler-echocardiographic variables. J Am Coll Cardiol 13:1613–1621
4 Sartori MP, Quinones MA, Kuo LC (1987) Relation of Doppler-derived left ventricular fill-

ing parameters to age and radius/thickness ratio in normal and pathologic states. Am J Cardiol 59:1179–1182

5 Stoddard MF, Pearson AC, Kern MJ, Ratcliff J, Mrosek DG, Labovitz AJ (1989) Left ventricular diastolic function: comparison of pulsed Doppler echocardiographic and hemodynamic indices in subjects with and without coronary disease. J Am Coll Cardioll 13:327–336

6 Konstadt SN, Reich DL, Thys DM, Hillel Z, Louie E (1990) Importance of atrial systole to ventricular filling redicted by transesophageal echocardiography. Anesthesiology 72:971–976

7 Humphrey LS, Stinson DC, Humphrey MJ, Finney RS, Zeller PA, Judd MR, Blanck TJJ (1990) Volatile anesthetic effects on left ventricular relaxation in swine. Anesthesiology 73:731–738

8 Housmans PR, Murat I (1988) Comparative effects of halothane, enflurane, and isoflurane at equipotent anesthetic concentrations on isolated ventricular myocardium of the ferret. II. Relaxation. Anesthesiology 69:464–471

9 Montoyo JR, Angel J, Valle V, Gausi C (1973) Cardioversion of tachycardias by transesophageal atrial pacing. Am J Cardiol 32:85–90

10 Benson DW Jr (1987) Transesophageal electrocardiography and cardiac pacing: state of the art. Circulation 75 [Suppl III]: 86–90

11 Waldo AL, Wells JL Jr, Cooper TB, MacLean WAH (1981) Temporary cardiac pacing: Application and techniques in the treatment of cardiac arrhythmias. Prog Cardiovasc Dis 23:451–474

12 Sterz H, Prager H, Koller H (1978) Transesophageal rapid stimulation of the left atrium in atrial tachycardia. Z Cardiol 67:136–138

13 Kerr C, Gallagher JJ, Smith WM, Sterba R, German LD, Cook L, Kassell JH (1983) The induction of atrial flutter and fibrillation and termination of atrial flutter by esophageal pacing. PACE 6: 60–72

14 Dunnigan A, Benson DW Jr, Benditt DG (1985) Atrial flutter in infancy: Diagnosis, clinical features, and treatment. Pediatrics 75: 725–729

15 Pattison CZ, Atlee JL, Mathews EL, Buljubasic N, Entress JJ (1991) Atrial pacing thresholds measured in anesthetized patients with the use of an esophageal stethoscope modified for pacing. Anesthesiology 74:854–859

16 Pattison CZ, Atlee JL, Krebs LH, Madireddi L, Kettler RE (1991) Transesophageal indirect atrial pacing for drug-resistant sinus bradycardia. Anesthesiology 74:1141–1144

17 Dreifus LS, Hessen SE (1990) Sinoatrial block: bradycardia-tachycardia syndrome. Learning Center highlights, vol 6 (49: American College of Cardiology, Bethesda, pp 1–4

18 Atlee JL, Bosnjak ZJ (1990) Mechanisms for cardiac dysrhythmias during anesthesia. Anesthesiology 72: 347–374

# Pacemaker Malfunction in Perioperative Settings

J. L. Atlee III

## Introduction

The permanent cardiac pacemaker, as opposed to temporary devices discussed in the previous chapter, is used for chronic management of patients with symptomatic bradycardia due to sinus node dysfunction or atrioventricular (AV) heart block [1]. Some newer permanent pacemakers may also incorporate special antitachycardia pacing modes.

There are an estimated 1 million patients world-wide with permanent pacemakers, with 500,000 of these in the United States [1, 2]. The great majority of these patients fit into the geriatric age category, but some are young adult or pediatric patients. With younger patients, pacing could be for symptomatic bradycardia following open heart surgery, inherited disorders affecting cardiac impulse formation or conduction, or for control of drug-refractory tachyarrhythmias.

Permanent cardiac pacemakers are highly sophisticated electronic devices. They incorporate complex electronic circuits for regulating the timing and delivery of pacing impulses, as well as for regulating and performing sensing functions. Additionally, most modern pacemakers are multiprogrammable rather than simple programmable (rate and output only), as was characteristic of older units. With such complexity, it should not be surprising that there is significant potential for pacemaker malfunction in perioperative settings, most of which can be attributed to improper programming, electrical or mechanical interference, or adverse pacemaker-patient interactions caused by the effects of drugs or imposed physiologic imbalance. Provided in this chapter is a brief review of modern pacemaker design and function, focusing on those aspects important to later discussion of types of pacemaker malfunction [3–7]. Then, from an anesthesiologist's perspective, I make recommendations for the perioperative management of pacemaker patients, with most emphasis on diagnosis of pacemaker malfunction and preventive management [8].

## Pacemaker Design and Function

In depth discussion of modern pacemaker design and function can be found in many of the other chapters of this book. In this section, a brief review of sorts, I describe in rather simple fashion modern pacemaker design and function, including provisions for physiologic pacing.

Permanent cardiac pacemakers provide electrical impulses to stimulate the heart, as well as electronic circuits for sensing and regulating the timing and current characteristics of stimuli. The pacemaker consists of a *pulse generator* ("can"), *electronic circuitry* for regulating current output, duration, timing, and sensing functions; and *leads* which connect the pulse generator to *electrodes* positioned on (epicardial) or within (endocardial) the heart. Electrodes may be *unipolar* or *bipolar*. With the former, the pacemaker "can" serves as the *anode,* and the myocardial electrode as the *cathode*. With the latter, both the anode and cathode are myocardial. Pulse generators weigh as little as 25 g and have a *battery* (lithium) *life* of up to 10 years. Finally, pacemakers may stimulate one (*single-chamber*) or both chambers (*dual-chamber*) of the heart.

The Inter-Society Commission for Heart Disease Resources (ICHD) has recommended a five-letter generic code to describe pacemaker function and pacing modalities (Table 1), [3]. For most purposes, the first three letters of this ICHD code can be used as shorthand notation to describe the pacing modes most commonly used to manage patients with bradycardia (Table 2). With *asynchronous pacing* (AOO, VOO,

**Table 1.** Inter-Society Commission for Heart Disease five-position pacemaker identification code

| I<br>Pacing | II<br>Sensing | III<br>Response | IV<br>Program | V<br>Antitachy |
|---|---|---|---|---|
| Atrium (A) | Atrium (A) | Inhibition (I) | Simple (S) | Bursts (B) |
| Ventricle (V) | Ventricle (V) | Triggering (T) | Multiple (M) | Normal (N)b |
| Dual (D) | Dual (D) | Both I and T (D) | Communicating (C) | Scanning (S)[c] |
|  | None (O) | None (O) | None (O) | External (E)[d] |
|  |  | Reverse (R)[a] |  | None (O) |

Positions I, II, and III indicate the chambers paced or sensed and the mode of response to sensed events, respectively. Positions IV and V indicate programming (Program) and special antitachycardia (Antitachy) features, respectively.
[a]pacemaker activates only at fast rates; [b]paces at normal rate when tachycardia is sensed; [c]provides scanning function such as timed extra stimuli throughout diastole; [d]antitachycardia function(s) activated by some external means (radiofrequency, magnet, other).

**Table 2.** Shorthand notation for common pacing modes

| ICHD code | Pacing mode |
|---|---|
| AOO, VOO, DOO | Asynchronous |
| AAI, VVI | Atrial, ventricular-inhibited (demand) |
| VAT | Atrial tracking |
| DVI, DDI | AV sequential |
| DDD | AV universal |

DOO), one or both chambers of the heart are paced without regard to native cardiac myopotentials; that is, no sensing function is provided. *Atrial-inhibited* (AAI) or *ventricular-inhibited* (VVI) *pacers* are inhibited by sensed atrial or ventricular myopotentials. An *atrial-tracking pacer* (VAT) paces the ventricle after each sensed atrial myopotential; that is, sensed P waves trigger ventricular output. In patients with normal sinus function, but with AV heart block, the VAT pacer preserves atrial transport function (discussed in the previons chapter). *AV sequential pacers* (DVI, DDI) also preserve atrial transport function. They pace one or both chambers, with ventricular or both atrial and ventricular stimulation inhibited following sensed myopotentials (DVI or DDI, respectively). With *AV universal pacers* (DDD), there can be sensing and pacing in both cardiac chambers. For example, the DDD pacer responds to sensed atrial myopotentials by inhibiting atrial output and triggering ventricular stimuli after some preset AV interval. With sensed ventricular myopotentials, on the other hand, there is inhibition of atrial and ventricular output for some programmed time (escape) interval. DVI and DDD pacers can be *committed* or *noncommitted.* With a committed pacer, there is inactivation of ventricular sensing during the programmed AV time interval. The pacer is therefore committed to deliver a ventricular stimulus after every atrial beat, regardless of whether spontaneous ventricular myopotentials occur during the programmed AV interval. Spontaneous ventricular myopotentials occurring outside the programmed AV interval, however, inhibit both atrial and ventricular pacer output. With the noncommitted pacer, there is ventricular sensing during the AV interval. However, to avoid ventricular sensing of atrial myopotentials or stimuli, which could inhibit ventricular output, the pacemaker can be programmed to provide a brief *blanking refractory period* (ventricular sensing amplifier only) during delivery of the atrial stimulus.

There is currently much interest on the part of implanting physicians and the pacemaker industry in providing more *physiologic pacing.* Requirements for this include proper *AV synchronization* to preserve atrial transport function and *rate responsiveness* to provide for increased physiologic needs of the body, as with exercise. The incorporation of technology to accomplish physiologic pacing further complicates any discussion of pacemaker design and function, as well as providing ample added opportunity for adverse effects of pacing and pacemaker malfunction (see below). Nonetheless, pacing with AV synchrony to preserve atrial transport function can be expected to alleviate symptoms of the pacemaker syndrome[1] and to improve cardiac performance in patients with poor ventricular diastolic function. In the patient without supraventricular tachyarrhythmias, but with normal sinus node function, the easiest way to accomplish rate-responsive pacing is to program a pacing mode which tracks atrial activity (VAT, DDI, DDD). In patients with supraventricular tachyarrhythmias, however, one-to-one tracking of P waves with ventricular stimuli could cause profound circulatory imbalance. In these patients, physiologic sensing devices are used for rate-responsive pacing. Such sensing devices might detect changes in temperature, pH, QT interval, or thoracic impedance, as discussed in other chapters.

[1]Symptoms of weakness, fatigue, dizziness, or near-syncope consequent to valvular regurgitation, hypotension caused by reflex peripheral vasodilation secondary to activation of stretch mechanoreceptors, or low cardiac output, all consequent to ventricular pacing with improper AV synchronization or retrograde atrial activation in patients with intact VA conduction.

Thus, provision for dual-chamber or physiologic pacing presents many possibilities for adverse effects of pacing, some of which are not strictly types of pacemaker malfunction. As already mentioned, atrial-tracking pacemakers may track supraventricular tachycardia on a one-to-one basis. Symptoms or signs of circulatory or coronary insufficiency from this can be somewhat alleviated by programming an upper rate limit for ventricular output. However, the problem can be altogether eliminated by using some other physiologic sensing modality. Ventricular electrodes might also sense atrial myopotentials or pacing artifacts, with resultant inhibition of ventricular output. This is referred to as *cross talk.* Cross talk is prevented by programming a short ventricular "blanking period" (above). Finally, atrial-tracking modes may be associated with pacemaker-mediated tachycardia ("endless-loop tachycardia"). For this to occur, there must be atrial sensing and the patient must have intact retrograde (VA) conduction. If so, the following might occur: (1) A premature junctional or ventricular beat is conducted back to the atria and sensed. (2) The sensed retrograde P wave, in turn, triggers a paced ventricular beat. (3) Paced ventricular beats are also conducted back to the ventricles. (4) The process keeps on repeating itself as a pacemaker-mediated tachycardia. Symptoms of a pacemaker-mediated tachycardia can be alleviated by programming an upper rate limit for ventricular output, or the problem can be prevented by programming appropriate atrial sensing refractory periods or using alternative pacing modes.

## Pacemaker Malfunction

Physicians who care for patients with pacemakers in the perioperative environment should be aware of some of the more important potential types of pacemaker malfunction. These include: (1) failure to pace; (2) failure to sense; (3) oversensing; and (4) pacing at an altered rate.

*Failure to Pace.* The failure to produce paced (capture) beats can be due to no stimulus being delivered or to failure of delivered stimuli to depolarize excitable myocardium. Lack of stimulation is most commonly caused by pulse generator component failure or power source (battery) depletion, but lead wire defects or fracture, cross talk (-above), or oversensing (below) can also be the cause. The failure to depolarize excitable myocardium is most commonly due to lead dislodgement or migration, defective leads (insulation defects, lead wire fracture), or to increased pacing thresholds (Table 3). Finally, it is important to recognize that failure to pace can easily be misdiagnosed if pacing stimuli are delivered during the myocardial refractory period.

**Table 3.** Causes for increased pacing thresholds

| |
|---|
| First 1–4 weeks following implantation |
| Acute physiologic imbalance (especially $K^+$) |
| Class 1 antiarrhythmic drugs (most if not all) |
| Local, but likely not inhalation or intravenous anesthetics |

*Failure to Sense.* Sensing failure is most commonly caused by lead dislodgement. Other causes include inadequate amplitude or distorted shape of sensed myopotentials. This could be secondary to the effects of disease, drugs, or metabolic imbalance; to inappropriate programming of sensing and related functions; to lead wire and connector defects; or to pulse generator component failure. The misdiagnosis of sensing failure is commonly made when spontaneous myopotentials coincide or fuse with pacing stimuli, or the pacemaker has reverted to asynchronous operation unbeknownst to the observer.

*Oversensing.* A pacemaker may detect signals other than the ones it is supposed to detect: oversensing. For example, ventricular sensing modes may sense T waves if the venticular sensing amplifier has been programmed with too much sensitivity or the ventricular sensing refractory period is too short. Unusually large T waves (hyperkalemia) or delayed ones (long QT interval, hypokalemia, or hypocalcemia) may also be the cause of ventricular oversensing. Furthermore, a dislodged ventricular electrode in the right ventricular outflow tract may sense atrial mypotentials as well as or instead of the ones it is supposed to detect.

Atrial sensing modes may sense ventricular mypotentials if the atrial signals are too small, which could result in the failure to initiate appropriate atrial refractory periods. Cross talk (above) and sensing of skeletal myopotentials leading to pacemaker inhibition are also examples of oversensing. Other examples of oversensing include detection of "make-break signals" from loose or fractured leads and pacemaker malfunction caused by electromagnetic interference (below). Oversensing is corrected by reprogramming the pacemaker or converting it to asynchronous operation.

*Pacing at an Altered Rate.* This can have several causes: (1) oversensing leading to inappropriate inhibition or triggering of output; (2) rate drift or reduction due to component aging or power source depletion; or (3) no stimulus output or pacing at an accelerated rate consequent to component failure. The latter, termed *runaway pacemaker,* is potentially the most lethal of pacemaker malfunctions. It has virtually been eliminated in current models of pacers by the incorporation of circuits limiting pacer output to typically less than 150 pulses/min. Nevertheless, if runaway pacemaker does occur, it is corrected by disconnecting the leads from the pulse generator and removing the device promptly. Magnet application usually has no effect to decrease the paced rate during runaway pacemaker.

The misdiagnosis of pacing at an altered rate is easily made if the pacemaker provides *rate hysteresis.* With hysteresis, the programmed *escape interval* (time the pacemaker waits to initiate pacing with bradycardia or asystole) is set longer than the *automatic interval* (the time between paced beats once pacing has commenced) to maximize the possibility of spontaneous rhythm. Pacing at an altered rate may be misdiagnosed if there is incorrect notation of programmed parameters in the patient's chart or nonpacemaker artifacts are misinterpreted by the observer as pacing spikes.

**Perioperative Management of the Pacemaker Patient**

Topics to be discussed relevant to the perioperative management of patients with pacemakers include: (1) preoperative evaluation of the patient; (2) electromagnetic interference; (3) myopotential inhibition; (4) competing rhythms; (5) patient transport and positioning; (6) pacing system analysis; and (7) management of pacemaker implantation.

*Patient Evaluation.* Patients with pacemakers are likely to have significant cardiovascular and other major organ system disease. It is important that there be a complete history and physical and that patients be carefully evaluated as to functional status, progression of disease, and current medications. Results of indicated diagnostic and laboratory tests (including a recent ECG and serum electrolytes) should be in the chart. It should be recognized by all that with the anticipation of anesthesia and surgery, and other perioperative stress, it is not uncommon for patients with demand pacemakers to have an adequate spontaneous rhythm. If so, the pacemaker will be suppressed and the casual observer not certain as to the functional status of the pacemaker. To ascertain proper pacemaker function, vagal maneuvres can be used to slow the rate of spontaneous rhythm. These could be with the Valsalva maneuver, carotid sinus massage, or the administration of edrophonium. The latter drug, a short-acting cholinesterase inhibitor with little negative inotropic effect, is administered intravenously (5 – 10 mg). If vagal maneuvers fail or are contraindicated, the ability of the pacemaker to provide cardiac stimulation can be established by interrogation of the pacemaker with a suitable pacing system analyzer (below), by converting the unit to asynchronous operation with an external magnet, or by reprogramming. Further concerning patient evaluation, it is necessary that the physician responsible for perioperative management of the pacemaker patient (usually the anesthesiologist) be aware of the indication(s) for pacing, as well as the programmed mode(s) of operation and time since implantation. This information should be found in the patient's medical records or on a pacemaker identification card carried by the patient. Finally, time permitting, preoperative consultation by a cardiologist or the implanting physician is always appropriate and preferred when possible.

*Electromagnetic Interference (EMI).* Diagnostic x-rays should not affect pacemaker function. Strong ionizing beams of radiation, nuclear magnetic resonance imaging, and surgical electrocautery are the most common sources of EMI likely to affect pacemaker function in perioperative settings. Although most demand pacemakers are designed to revert to asynchronous operation in the presence of *continuous* EMI from any source, this may not be so with *intermittent* or *modulating EMI*. The latter might temporarily inhibit pulse generator output, producing periods of bradycardia or asystole. The following precautions can help to reduce the risk of adverse effects to the patient from pacemaker malfunction caused by EMI: (1) Use bipolar electrocautery if possible. (2) If unipolar electrocautery is to be used, position the grounding plate as far as possible from the pulse generator. (3) Monitor pulse pressure (e.g., pulse oximetry, direct arterial pressure monitoring) or heart sounds continuously to detect inhibition of pacemaker output. (4) If pacemaker inhibition becomes a problem, convert the unit to asynchronous operation by reprogramming it or with a magnet.[2] (5) Shield the pulse generator from direct ionizing beams of radiation. (6) Do not position defibrillation or cardioversion paddles or pads directly over the pulse generator, use only the lowest possible energies for electroversion, and have the pacemaker checked for proper function following cardioversion or defibrillation.

*Myopotential Inhibition.* Skeletal myopotentials from various causes, including respiratory excursions with mechanical ventilation, succinylcholine-induced fasciculations, seizures, or direct muscle stimulation, could be sensed by some pacemakers, leading to inappropriate inhibition or triggering of output. This is more likely to be a problem with unipolar devices, where the pacemaker can (anode) provides a large-surface-area electrode for sensing myopotentials. One should carefully monitor the pulse and ECG for detection of myopotential inhibition. If myopotential inhibition causes circulatory insufficiency, the pacemaker should be reprogrammed to asynchronous operation.

*Competing Rhythmus.* Because the current output from pacemakers is relatively small, the risk of inducing malignant ventricular tachyarrhythmias by a stimulus falling on the T wave is small, except possibly under the following circumstances: (1) significant acid-base, electrolyte, or other physiologic imbalance; (2) drug-induced susceptibility (e.g., digitalis excess, high catecholamine concentrations); and (3) impaired myocardial oxygenation, especially with coronary insufficiency or in the setting of acute myocardial infarction.

*Patient Transport and Positioning.* Care must be taken when transporting or positioning patients with temporary transvenous pacing leads to prevent accidental electrode dislodgement or perforation of the ventricle. While electrode dislodgement or perforation is not likely to be a problem with leads inserted by the subclavian route, it can be with leads inserted by most other transvenous routes if there is flexion or extension of the affected extremity or neck. During patient transport, the external pulse generator should be accessible, the ECG and pulse or heart sounds monitored, and chronotopic drugs available for management of bradycardic arrhythmias. Additionally, it is recommended that latex gloves be worn when handling temporary pacing leads to protect the patient from microshock.

*Pacing System Analysis.* It is possible that the physician caring for the pacemaker patient might be asked to use a pacing system analyzer during implantation or revision of a permanent pacing system. The analyzer should be matched by manufacturer with the system being analyzed, as with programming devices. Otherwise, it could provide grossly misleading results. Pacing system analysis can provide information concerning pulse generator output, pacing thresholds, lead impedance, amplitude and slew

---

[2]Reprogramming may be preferred since an external magnet placed over the pulse generator in the presence of intermittent EMI could lead to reprogramming of some pacemakers, but only if the programming sequence requires both magnet activation and transfer of programming information by radiofrequency signals.

rate of sensed myopotentials, and other functions. Ideally, the implanting physician should be responsible for and direct any use of a pacing system analyzer.

*Pacemaker Implantation.* Most permanent pacing systems today employ transvenous (endocardial) leads. These and the pulse generator are usually implanted using local or regional anesthesia. The use of general anesthesia has been discouraged, possibly since some believe anesthetic drugs do affect pacing thresholds and sensing function (yet to be conclusively shown), and also to what I know is a widely held but perhaps incorrect notion – namely, that many pacemaker patients are too sick to tolerate a general anesthetic. Perhaps we should reconsider the advice regarding use of general anesthesia in view of significant advances in anesthetic and monitoring practice, so that today patients with severely compromised myocardial function can be safely anesthetized with drugs that have little effect on cardiac electrophysiologic or mechanical function. I hold this view because I am convinced that a well-managed general anesthetic can be less stressful for patients, and can also provide more nearly ideal operating conditions and more time for the implanting physician to complete his task. If general anesthesia is to be used, however, a functioning temporary pacing system should be in place. This is because chronotropic drugs cannot be relied upon to improve ventricular conduction or augment the rate of secondary pacemakers. In fact, such drugs may cause unstable escape rhythms or quite troublesome ventricular tachyarrhythmias.

## References


1 Frye RL, Collins JJ, DeSanctis RW, Dodge HT, Dreifus LS, Fisch C, Geths LS, Gillette PC, Parsonnet V, Reeves J et al. (1984) Guidelines for permanent cardiac pacemaker implantation. Circulation 70: 331A–339A

2 Zipes DP, Duffin EG (1988) Cardiac pacemakers. In: Braunwald E (ed) Heart disease, 3rd edn. Saunders, Philadelphia, pp 717–741

3 Parsonnet V, Furman S, Smyth NPD, Bilitch M (1983) Optimal resources for implantable cardiac pacemakers. Circulation 68: 224A–244A

4 Furman S, Hayes DL, Holmes DR Jr (1986) A practice of pacing. Futura, Mount Kisco, pp 1–16, 27–73, 75–95, 219–251, 305–331

5 Kugler JD, Danford DA (1989) Pacemakers in children: an update. Am Heart J 117:665–679

6 Manolis AS, Rastegar H, Estes NAM III (1989) Automatic implantable cardioverter defibrillator. Current status. JAMA 262:1362–1368

7 Platia EV (1987) Management of cardiac arrhythmias. The nonpharmacologic approach. Lippincott, Philadelphia, pp 156–218, 272–303

8 Atlee JL (1990) Perioperative cardiac dysrhythmias, 2nd edn. Year Book, Chicago, pp 162–176, 318–321, 323–325, 328–332

# Guidelines for the Perioperative Management of Pacemaker and Automatic Internal Cardioverter-Defibrillator Patients

K.H Tscheliessnigg, H. Gombotz, and J.L. Atlee III

## Introduction

Electrical treatment for bradyarrhythmias in the form of permanently implanted pacemakers is now an established therapeutic modality. Incorporation of antitachycardia pacing modes into pacemakers and the introduction of the automatic internal cardioverter-defibrillator (AICD) represent more recent advances. Therefore, larger numbers of patients with implanted electrical devices for treatment of brady- or tachyarrhythmias can be expected to undergo surgical or diagnostic procedures requiring anesthesia or monitored anesthesia care. Additionally, as pacemakers become more and more complex, with incorporation of increasing numbers of programmable functions as well as provision for rate adaptive pacing, there appears to be increased potential for adverse interactions and malfunction in electrically contaminated hospital environments. In this chapter, we offer more specific guidelines for perioperative management of patients with pacemakers or antitachycardia devices. These "consensus" recommendations are based on the editor's perspective of information presented in previous chapters.

## Perioperative Pacemaker and AICD Malfunction

Pacemaker and AICD malfunction should always be anticipated and often occurs during medical or surgical diagnostic and therapeutic interventions, for any of the following reasons:

1. Device malfunction due to spontaneous or induced arrhythmias, incorrect programming, competing rhythms, or power source (battery) depletion.
2. Physical damage to the pacemaker system or AICD, including thermal damage to pulse generator, mechanical damage to or disruption of pacemaker leads and electrodes, or electrode dislodgement produced by shockwaves of a lithotripter.
3. Increase in pacing, cardioversion, or defibrillation thresholds produced by acute changes in acid-base or electrolyte balance (especially potassium), myocardial ischemia or infarction, or the effects of antiarrhythmic or other drugs used in perioperative settings.
4. Direct or indirect effects of electromagnetic interference, especially that produced by surgical electrocautery devices, ionizing beams of radiation, and nuclear magnetic resonance imaging.

*Device malfunction.* Properly functioning pacemakers or AICD should continue to function well throughout the perioperative period. Some precautions can help assure this. In addition to routine preoperative patient evaluation, the patient's dependence on the device must be ascertained and the system evaluated for proper function. This is especially indicated for patients who have not had their systems evaluated in the recent past (6 months to 1 year) or who present with symptoms or signs of system malfunction or failure. Indications for implantation of the device, time of implantation, type of system, manufacturer, and programmed modes of operation for pacemakers should all be determined. For most patients, this information will be found in the medical records or on a pacemaker identification card carried by the patient.

In many patients, thorough clinical examination, chest X-ray, and surface ECG (possibly, 24-h Holter ECG) are sufficient to detect pacemaker malfunction. The degree of patient dependency on the pacemaker can be assessed by programming the device to its slowest available rate or by transiently inhibiting it. This may be necessary because many patients will be in spontaneous rhythm when facing diagnostic or surgical procedures. In these patients, the ability of the pacemaker to function as intended can be tested with vagal maneuvers to slow the spontaneous rate. If this fails, the ability of the pacemaker to deliver pacing stimuli must be determined by converting the pulse generator to an asynchronous mode of pacing, either by reprogramming the device or with a magnet. In other patients, especially those with more complex pacing systems, a pacing system analyzer that is matched by the manufacturer to the specific pacemaker will be required to adequately evaluate pacemaker function. Finally, if the patient has an unfamiliar type or model of pacemaker, the manufacturer should be consulted for advice regarding possible adverse interactions in the hospital environment, as well as specific guidelines for indicated preventive or corrective perioperative management.

*Physical Damage of System.* Lead dislodgement, myocardial perforation due to electrode migration, lead insulation defects, and lead wire fracture are the most common causes for loss of atrial or ventricular sensing or the failure to capture. Physical damage to leads could result from overstretching during patient transport or positioning, with spontaneous patient movements, during mechanical ventilation [1], or due to mishandling of leads, electrodes, or tissues in close proximity to these. Direct or close contact between the electrocautery probe tip and the pulse generator may produce local heating. This could damage the pulse generator circuitry or myocardial tissue at the electrode interface. Damage to myocardial tissue could result in increased pacing thresholds. Also, with electrocautery performed close to pacemaker leads or electrodes, there is the danger of microshock to the patient with resulting arrhythmias or ventricular fibrillation. For these reasons, if the pacemaker system is within or close to the contemplated surgical or irradiated fields, consideration should be given to explantation of the pacing system and provision of some means for temporary pacing.

*Increase in Pacing Cardioversion, or Defibrillation Thresholds.* Myocardial thresholds for electrical stimulation may be altered by many factors. However, it does not appear that pacing thresholds are significantly altered by inhalation anesthetics [2]. They may be elevated by drugs including class 1 antiarrhythmics and local anesthetics

[3], acute potassium imbalance [4], and myocardial ischemia or infarction. While infarcted or fibrosed tissue cannot be stimulated, it is able to conduct current from the tip of the pacemaker electrode. As a result, the surface area of the electrode is enlarged so that delivered current density decreases. This can eventually lead to loss of capture. Effective pacing can then only be reestablished by increasing pacemaker output.

*Effects of Electromagnetic Interference (EMI).* Diagnostic X-rays, ultrasonography, and laser surgery should not affect pacemaker function, but, as discussed earlier in this book and elsewhere, electrocautery, nerve stimulators, transurethral resection, radiation therapy, lithotripsy, and nuclear magnetic resonance imaging can interfere with pacemaker function [5–10]. During exposure to continuous EMI, regardless of source, most pacemakers will revert to an asynchronous mode of pacing. Following cessation of continuous EMI, however, there should be restoration of the previously programmed parameters of operation. This may not be the case with intermittent or modulating EMI, which could be sensed as native myocardial activity with inhibition of pacemaker output consequent to this. However, intermittent EMI is more likely to be sensed by unipolar than by bipolar pacemakers. The reason for this is that the large interelectrode distance produces an antenna effect and encourages sensing of extrinsic or intrinsic EMI (e.g., skeletal muscle myopotentials) at the anode (pacemaker can). Despite preventive measures, including proper shielding, electronic filtering of extraneous signals, and provision of an interference mode, unipolar pacemakers can still have a lot of problems with differentiating native myocardial from extraneous signals or other interference. Coating of the titanium or stainless steel pulse generator housing with silicone or polyurethane can nevertheless prevent direct intrusion of EMI. Even so, during therapeutic irradiation, it is necessary to protect the pulse generator and its component circuitry with proper external shielding. If this is not feasible for other reasons, then the pacemaker will have to be explanted temporarily and provision for some means of temporary pacing made during radiation therapy treatments. Alternatively, it may be practical to reimplant the pacemaker pulse generator well outside the irradiated field.

Finally, following any exposure to EMI, pacemaker function must be assessed carefully. The same is true for AICD or other antitachycardia devices, even though the latter devices should have been deactivated before any exposure to strong extrinsic EMI sources, including those discussed above for pacemakers.

## Specific Guidelines for Management

*EMI from Surgical Electrocautery.* Ideally, bipolar electrocautery devices should be used for all pacemaker patients to reduce the potential for pacemaker malfunction during exposure to electrocautery EMI. However, if unipolar electrocautery must be used, the grounding plate should be as far as possible from the pulse generator to reduce susceptibility to inhibition by sensed EMI [11]. With older, simple programmable (rate and output only) models of demand pacemakers, it was a common and acceptable practice to convert the device to asynchronous operation by placing a strong magnet over the pulse generator. With newer, multiprogrammable pulse generators, it is strongly recommended that the pulse generator be programmed to asynchronous or synchronous (demand) operation. The reason for this is that with some models of pacemakers, the "read-only" window (pacemaker receptive to programming information) may require opening by a magnet, even though radiofrequency commands are used for programming. If so, random or "phantom" reprogramming is possible during exposure to EMI from electrocautery [7]. With other newer models of pacemakers, a special mode, similar to noninvasive pacing threshold testing, may be triggered by application of a magnet. Therefore, we reiterate that *with modern programmable pacemakers, a magnet should not be placed over the pulse generator during any exposure to EMI*. Rather, the pulse generator should be programmed to an asynchronous or demand mode of operation (Table 1). If the patient would not be at increased risk from competitive pacing (i.e., a patient with acute electrolyte or other physiologic imbalance, digitalis toxicity, or receiving circulatory support with inotropic or chronotropic drugs, etc.), an asynchronous pacing mode is acceptable or even preferred. However, if the patient is possibly at increased risk with competive pacing, and especially if not pacemaker-dependent (i.e., has adequate spontaneous rhythm most of the time) then some mode of demand pacing is preferred.

For all patients with programmable or rate-responsive pacemakers, appropriate (matched by manufacturer) pacing system analyzers and programming devices, as well as a trained operator, should be in the vicinity and available during patient exposure to EMI, just in case the patient becomes endangerd by pacemaker malfunction or competing rhythms. However, a trained operator may not be immediately available. In that case, we point out that all programming devices contain a trouble-shooting or "panic button" which will reprogram a malfunctioning device to an output of 5 V and rate of 70 paced pulses per minute in the ventricular-inhibited mode. Finally, an external cardioverter-defibrillator and suitable external temporary pacing device should be available at a moment's notice.

**Table 1.** Recommendations for reprogramming pacemakers in patients who will be exposed to surgical electrocautery

| *Mode of Pacing* | *Pacemaker-dependent* | *Non-pacer-dependent* |
|---|---|---|
| Fixed rate (AOO, VOO, DOO) | Leave AOO, VOO, DOO | Not applicable |
| Demand, single-chamber (AAI, VVI) | Program AOO, VOO | Leave AAI, VVI |
| Demand, dual-chamber (VAT, VDD, DVI, DDD) | Program VOO, DOO | Program VVI, DVI |
| Rate-responsive (AAIR, VVIR, DDDR) | Program AOO, VOO, DOO | Program AAI, VVI, DDD |
| Antitachycardia | Deactivate | Deactivate |
| AICD | Deactivate | Deactivate |

*Radiation Therapy, Nuclear Magnetic Resonance Imaging.* Our recommendation for reprogramming pacemakers when surgical electrocautery is to be used also apply to radiation therapy or nuclear magnetic resonance imaging. Also, during exposure to ionizing radiation, the pulse generator should be adequately shielded. For additional precautions, the pacemaker manufacturer and earlier chapters dealing with these two special circumstances should be consulted. Pacemaker function should always be checked following these procedures

*Cardioversion and Defibrillation (Electroversion).* Pacemakers may be reprogrammed or destroyed during electroversion [12, 13]. Paddles or disposable electrode pads used for electroversion should be positioned as far as possible away from the pulse generator, and also not directly over or in line with implanted pacemaker leads. Thus, the anteroposterior as opposed to anterolateral paddle or electrode pad position is preferred for most pacemaker patients. Only the lowest possible energies should be used for shocks, and the ability of the pacemaker to function should be checked following electroversion.

*Myopotential Inhibition.* Myopotentials, whether generated by voluntary or involuntary muscle movements (e.g., succinylcholine-induced muscle fasciculations, seizure disorders, direct muscle stimulation, shivering, large respiratory excursions with mechanical ventilators), can produce pacemaker inhibition if myopotentials have sufficient amplitude or slew rates to be sensed as intracardiac signals [1, 14, 15]. Inhibition will be more a problem with unipolar than with bipolar electrode systems. If myopotential inhibition becomes apparent and is hemodynamically or otherwise significant, consider reprogramming the pacemaker to an asynchronous mode of operation — but only if competing rhythms will pose no threat to the patient. Otherwise, reprogram the ventricular sensing amplifier so that larger R or S waves must be sensed to inhibit pulse generator output.

*Antitachycardia Pacemakers and AICD.* EMI from any source may cause an AICD device to discharge inappropriately or initiate an antitachycardia pacing sequence with antitachycardia pacemakers. Newer models of antitachycardia pacemakers may incorporate AICD backup. With these devices, at least in theory, sensed EMI might initiate antitachycardia pacing followed by internal electroversion shocks. Therefore, *it is recommended that AICD and antitachycardia pacemakers be deactivated before exposure to electrocautery,* and probably also before radiation therapy unless evidence to the contrary is presented.

Magnets and pacing system analyzers or programming devices should be kept away from AICD pulse generators because of possible activation, deactivation, or inhibition [16]. Nuclear magnetic resonance imaging can also produce damage to or activate an AICD device, and therefore should be avoided.

Adverse interactions between pacemakers and AICD in patients with both devices have been reported (Table 2) [17]. If temporary perioperative pacing is required for a patient with an AICD, the AICD should first be deactivated. If a permanent pacemaker is to be implanted in a patient with an AICD, a bipolar electrode system should be used. Only the lowest possible pulse amplitude and highest R-wave sensitivity should

**Table 2.** Adverse interactions between pacemakers and AICD in patients with both devices

| |
|---|
| 1. Pacing stimulus interpreted as normal QRS in patient with ventricular fibrillation causes failure to deliver shocks. |
| 2. Pacemaker sensing failure with extrastimulation leads to interpretation of pacing stimuli and QRS complexes by AICD as ventricular fibrillation, causing delivery of inappropriate shocks. |
| 3. Sufficient delay between the pacing stimulus artefact and the resulting R wave produces double counting, which leads to inappropriate AICD discharge. |
| 4. Programming of pacemaker may cause the AICD to discharge inappropriately. |

be programmed. Further, only physiologic pacing rates should be programmed, and these must be lower than the AICD activation rate.

When AICD patients require surgical or diagnostic procedures, anesthetic management must be appropriate for the patient's general medical condition. The AICD will be deactivated during the procedure so that if the patient requires electroversion, external paddles or electrode pads will have to be used. Only the lowest possible energy shocks should be used to avoid permanent damage to the AICD pulse generator. If myocardial patch electrodes have been implanted with the AICD, then the external defibrillation paddles or electrode pads should be oriented perpendicular to a line drawn between the two myocardial patch electrodes. In this way, electroversion energy can pass directly from the chest wall to the myocardium. Finally, when caring for patients with activated AICD devices, latex surgical gloves should be worn. Without the protection afforded by gloves, static charges could produce inappropriate AICD discharge, especially during cardiopulmonary resuscitation.

## References

1 Thiagarajah S, Azar I, Agres M, Lear E (1983) Pacemaker malfunction associated with positive-pressure ventilation. Anesthesiology 58: 565–566
2 Zaidan JR, Curling PE, Craver JM (1985) Effect of enflurane, isoflurane and halothane on pacing stimulation thresholds in man. PACE 8: 32–34
3 Preston TA, Judge RD (1969) Alteration of pacemaker thresholds by drug and physiological factors. Ann NY Acad Sci 167: 686–692
4 O'Reilly MV, Murnaghan DP, Williams MB (1974) Transvenous pacemakers failure induced by hyperkalemia. JAMA 228: 336–337
5 Levine Pa, Balady GJ, Lazar HL, Belott PH, Roberts AJ (1986) Electrocautery and pacemakers: Management of the paced patient subject to electrocautery. Ann Thorac Surg 41: 313–317
6 Lerner SM (1973) Suppression of a demand pacemaker by transurethral electrocautery. Anesth Analg 52: 703–706
7 Domino KB, Smith TC (1983) Electrocautery-induced reprogramming of a pacemaker using a precordial magnet. Anesth Analg 62: 609–612
8 Shaprio WA, Roizen MF, Singleton MA, Morady F, Bainto CR, Gaynor RL (1985) Intraoperative pacemaker complications. Anesthesiology 63: 319–322
9 Belott PH, Sands S, Warren J (1984) Resetting of DDD pacemakers due to EMI. PACE 7: 169–172

10 Rasmussen MJ, Hayes DL, Vlietstra RE, Thorsteinsson G (1988) Can transcutaneous nerve stimulation be safely used in patients with permanent cardiac pacemakers? Mayo Clin Proc 63: 443–445
11 Simon AB (1977) Perioperative management of the pacemaker system. Anesthesiology 46: 127–131
12 Levine PA, Barold SS, Fletcher RL, Talbot P (1983) Adverse acute and chronic effects of electrical defibrillation and cardioversion on implanted unipolar pacemaker systems. J Am Coll Cardiol 6: 1413–1422
13 Barold SS, Ong L, Scovil J, Heinle R, Wright TH (1978) Reprogramming of implanted pacemaker following external defibrillation. PAC E 1: 514–520
14 Gialafos J, Maillis A, Kalogeropoulos C, Kalikazaros J, Basiakos L, Avgoustakis D (1985) Inhibition of demand pacemakers by myopotentials. Am Heart J 109: 984–991
15 Lau CP, Linker NJ, Butrons GS, Ward DE, Camm AJ (1989) Myopotential interference in unipolar rate responsive pacemakers. PACE 12: 1324–1330
16 Gottlieb C, Miller JM, Rosenthal ME, Marchlinski FE (1988) Automatic implantable defibrillator discharge resulting from routine pacemaker programming. PACE 11: 336–338
17 Calkins H, Brinker J, Veltri EP, Guarnieri T, Levine JH (1990) Clinical interactions between pacemakers and automatic implantable cardioverter-defibrillator. J Am Coll Cardiol 16: 666–673

# Subject Index

Printing: Saladruck, Berlin
Binding: Buchbinderei Lüderitz & Bauer, Berlin